Drugs for Parasitic Infections

Published by

The Medical Letter, Inc.
145 Huguenot Street Suite 312
New Rochelle, New York 10801

800-211-2769
www.medicalletter.org

3rd Edition

(ISBN 978-0-9815278-7-1)

The Medical Letter Inc.
145 Huguenot Street Suite 312
New Rochelle, New York 10801

Contents

Introduction

With increasing travel, immigration, use of immunosuppressive drugs and the spread of HIV, physicians anywhere may see infections caused by parasites. The tables that follow list first-choice and alternative drugs for most parasitic infections. The principal adverse effects of these drugs are listed on pages 67–77. The table that begins on page 78 summarizes the known prenatal risks of antiparasitic drugs. The brand names and manufacturers of the drugs are listed on pages 83–86.

ACANTHAMOEBA keratitis

Drug of choice: Keratitis is typically associated with contact lens use.[1] A topical biguanide, 0.02% chlorhexidine or polyhexamethylene biguanide (PHMB, 0.02%), either alone or combined with a diamidine, propamidine isethionate *(Brolene)* or hexamidine *(Desomodine)*, have been used successfully.[2] They are administered hourly (or alternating every half hour) day and night for the first 48 hours and then continued on a reduced schedule for days to months.[3] None of these drugs is commercially available or approved for use in the US, but they can be obtained from compounding pharmacies. Leiter's Park Avenue Pharmacy, San Jose, CA (800-292-6773; www.leiterrx.com) is a compounding pharmacy that specializes in ophthalmic drugs. Expert Compounding Pharmacy, 6744 Balboa Blvd., Lake Balboa, CA 91406 (800-247-9767) and Medical Center Pharmacy, New Haven, CT (203-688-7064) are also compounding pharmacies. Other compounding pharmacies may be found through the National Association of Compounding Pharmacies (800-687-7850) or the Professional Compounding Centers of America (800-331-2498, www.pccarx.com). Propamidine is available over the counter in the UK and Australia. Hexamidine is available in France. Debridement is most useful during the stage of corneal epithelial infection; keratoplasty in medically unresponsive keratitis was successful in 31 eyes in 30 patients.[4] Most cysts are resistant to neomycin; its use is no longer recommended. Azole antifungal drugs (ketoconazole, itraconazole) have been used as oral or topical adjuncts. Successful treatment with topical or oral voriconazole has been reported in a small number of patients who had failed PHMB, chlorhexidine and hexamidine.[5,6] Use of corticosteroids is controversial. Prolonged therapy (≥6 months) may be necessary.[2]

1. FR Carvalho et al, Cornea 2009; 28:516.
2. JK Dart et al, Am J Ophthalmol 2009; 148:487.
3. GS Visvesvara, Curr Opin Infect Dis 2010; 23:590.
4. AS Kitzmann et al, Ophthalmology 2009; 116: 864.
5. BS Bang et al, Am J Ophthalmol 2010; 149:66.
6. EY Tu et al, Cornea 2010; 29:1066.

AMEBIASIS *(Entamoeba histolytica)*

	Drug	Adult dosage	Pediatric dosage
Asymptomatic			
Drug of choice:	Iodoquinol[1]	650 mg PO tid x 20d	30-40 mg/kg/d (max 2g) PO in 3 doses x 20d
OR	Paromomycin[2]	25-35 mg/kg/d PO in 3 doses x 7d	25-35 mg/kg/d PO in 3 doses x 7d
OR	Diloxanide furoate[3]*	500 mg PO tid x 10d	20 mg/kg/d PO in 3 doses x 10d
Mild to moderate intestinal disease			
Drug of choice:[4]	Metronidazole	500-750 mg PO tid x 7-10d	35-50 mg/kg/d PO in 3 doses x 7-10d
OR	Tinidazole[5]	2 g once PO daily x 3d	≥3yrs: 50 mg/kg/d (max 2g) PO in 1 dose x 3d
	either followed by		
	Iodoquinol[1]	650 mg PO tid x 20d	30-40 mg/kg/d (max 2g) PO in 3 doses x 20d
OR	Paromomycin[2]	25-35 mg/kg/d PO in 3 doses x 7d	25-35 mg/kg/d PO in 3 doses x 7d
Severe intestinal and extraintestinal disease			
Drug of choice:	Metronidazole	750 mg PO (or IV) tid x 7-10d	35-50 mg/kg/d PO (or IV) in 3 doses x 7-10d
OR	Tinidazole[5]	2 g once PO daily x 5d	≥3yrs: 50 mg/kg/d (max 2g) PO in 1 dose x 5d
	either followed by		
	Iodoquinol[1]	650 mg PO tid x 20d	30-40 mg/kg/d (max 2g) PO in 3 doses x 20d
OR	Paromomycin[2]	25-35 mg/kg/d PO in 3 doses x 7d	25-35 mg/kg/d PO in 3 doses x 7d

* Availability problems. See table of manufacturers on pages 83-86.

1. Iodoquinol should be taken after meals.

(continued)

AMEBIASIS (continued)

2. Paromomycin should be taken with a meal.
3. Not available commercially. It may be obtained through compounding pharmacies such as Expert Compounding Pharmacy, 6744 Balboa Blvd, Lake Balboa, CA 91406 (800-247-9767) or Medical Center Pharmacy, New Haven, CT (203-688-7064). Other compounding pharmacies may be found through the National Association of Compounding Pharmacies (800-687-7850) or the Professional Compounding Centers of America (800-331-2498, www.pccarx.com).
4. Nitazoxanide may be effective against a variety of protozoan and helminth infections (DA Bobak, Curr Infect Dis Rep 2006; 8:91; E Diaz et al, Am J Trop Med Hyg 2003; 68:384). It is effective against mild to moderate amebiasis, 500 mg PO bid x 3d (JF Rossignol et al, Trans R Soc Trop Med Hyg 2007; 101:1025; AE Escobedo et al, Arch Dis Child 2009; 94:478), but perhaps less so than metronidazole (S Becker et al, Am J Trop Hyg 2011; 84:581). Nitazoxanide is FDA-approved only for treatment of diarrhea caused by *Giardia* or *Cryptosporidium* (Med Lett Drugs Ther 2003; 45:29). It is available in 500-mg tablets and an oral suspension and should be taken with food.
5. A nitroimidazole similar to metronidazole, tinidazole appears to be as effective as metronidazole and better tolerated (Med Lett Drugs Ther 2004; 46:70). It should be taken with food to minimize GI adverse effects. For children and patients unable to take tablets, a pharmacist can crush the tablets and mix them with cherry syrup (*Humco*, and others). The syrup suspension is good for 7 days at room temperature and must be shaken before use (HB Fung and TL Doan, Clin Ther 2005; 27:1859). Ornidazole, a similar drug, is also used outside the US.

AMEBIC MENINGOENCEPHALITIS, primary and granulomatous[1]

	Drug	Adult dosage	Pediatric dosage
Primary Amebic Meningoencephalitis (PAM) – *Naegleria fowleri*[2,3]			
Drug of choice:	Amphotericin B (conventional formulation)[4]	0.25 mg/kg IV over 4-6 h. If tolerated, 0.5 mg/kg IV the following day, increasing to 1.5 mg/kg IV once/d as tolerated (max 1.5 mg/kg/day)	0.25 mg/kg IV over 4-6 h. If tolerated, 0.5 mg/kg IV the following day, increasing to 1.5 mg/kg IV once/d as tolerated (max 1.5 mg/kg/day)
	or	1 mg/kg IV once/d plus 0.5 mg/d intraventricularly (can start with 0.025-0.050 mg/d and increase to 0.5 mg/d)[5] (max 1.5 mg/kg once/d total dosage by both IV and intraventricular routes)	1 mg/kg IV once/d plus 0.5 mg/d intraventricularly (can start with 0.025-0.050 mg/d and increase to 0.5 mg/d)[5] (max 1.5 mg/kg once/d total dosage by both IV and intraventricular routes)
	Rifampin	10 mg/kg IV once/d (max 600 mg/d)	10 mg/kg IV once/d (max 600 mg/d)
	Fluconazole	12 mg/kg IV once/d	12 mg/kg IV once/d
	Azithromycin	500 mg IV once/d	20 mg/kg IV once/d (max 500 mg/d)
Granulomatous Amebic Encephalitis (GAE) – *Acanthamoeba* spp.[6-8]			
	Pentamidine[9]	4 mg/kg IV once/d	4 mg/kg IV once/d
	Sulfadiazine	1.5 g q6h PO	200 mg/kg/d PO in 4-6 doses (max 6 g/d)
	Flucytosine	37.5 mg/kg PO q6h (max 150 mg/kg/d)	37.5 mg/kg PO q6h (max 150 mg/kg/d)
	Fluconazole	12 mg/kg IV once/d	12 mg/kg IV once/d

(continued)

AMEBIC MENINGOENCEPHALITIS, primary and granulomatous (continued)

Infection	Drug	Adult dosage	Pediatric dosage
	Miltefosine[10]	<45 kg: 100 mg/d PO in 2 doses ≥45 kg: 150 mg/d PO in 3 doses	2.5 mg/kg/d PO in 2 doses (max 100 mg/d)
Granulomatous Amebic Encephalitis (GAE) – *Balamuthia mandrillaris*[11-16]			
	Azithromycin	500 mg IV once/d	20 mg/kg IV once/d (max 500 mg/d)
	Clarithromycin	14 mg/kg/d PO in 2 doses (max 2 g/d)	14 mg/kg/d PO in 2 doses (max 2 g/d)
	Pentamidine[9] Sulfadiazine	4 mg/kg IV once/d 1.5 g PO q6h	4 mg/kg IV once/d 200 mg/kg/d PO in 4-6 doses (max 6 g/d)
	Flucytosine	37.5 mg/kg PO q6h (max 150 mg/kg/d)	37.5 mg/kg PO q6h (max 150 mg/kg/d)
	Fluconazole	12 mg/kg IV once/d	12 mg/kg IV once/d
	Miltefosine[10]	<45 kg: 100 mg/d PO in 2 doses ≥45 kg: 150 mg/d PO in 3 doses	2.5 mg/kg/d PO in 2 doses (max 100 mg/d)

1. Meningoencephalitis caused by the free-living amebae *Naegleria fowleri*, *Acanthamoeba* spp., and *Balamuthia mandrillaris* has a mortality rate of >90%; effective treatment has not been established. Treatment recommendations are based on case reports of survivors, animal studies, and *in vitro* drug testing. Treatment decisions must be tailored to the clinical situation of each patient. Diagnostic assistance, specimen collection guidance, shipping instructions, and treatment recommendations are available through the CDC Emergency Operations Center at 770-488-7100.
2. JS Seidel et al, N Engl J Med 1982; 306:346.
3. J Vargas-Zepeda et al, Arch Med Res 2005; 36:83.

4. Although liposomal amphotericin B crosses the blood-brain barrier better than conventional amphotericin, it has been found to be less effective against primary amebic meningoencephalitis (PAM) caused by *Naegleria fowleri* in mice. Amphotericin B methyl ester was also found to be less effective in the mouse model (FL Schuster and GS Visvesvara, Int J Parasitol 2004; 34:1001). Because of the extremely poor prognosis of PAM due to *Naegleria fowleri*, aggressive treatment, including the use of intraventricular amphotericin, should be considered.
5. SW Chapman et al. In: Kauffman C, ed. Essentials of Clinical Mycology. 2nd ed. New York: Springer; 2011:41-55.
6. Immunocompromised patients with cutaneous acanthamoebiasis have been successfully treated with (1) pentamidine, flucytosine, and azithromycin in combination with topical chlorhexidine and 2% ketoconazole cream (S Oliva et al, South Med J 1999; 92:55); (2) pentamidine in combination with topical chlorhexidine and 2% ketoconazole cream followed by oral itraconazole (CA Slater et al, N Engl J Med 1994, 331:85); and (3) amphotericin B lipid complex and voriconazole (R Walia et al, Transplant Soc 2007; 9:51). Miltefosine, both oral and topical, has also shown success in treating cutaneous disease (AC Aichelburg et al, Emerg Infect Dis 2008; 14:1743; J Walochnik et al, J Antimicrob Chemother 2009; 64:539).
7. AC Aichelburg et al, Emerg Infect Dis 2008;14:1743.
8. M Seijo Martinez et al, J Clinical Microbiol 2000; 38:3892.
9. Addition of pentamidine is based on clinical judgement. Although it has good amebacidal activity *in vitro* and has been used successfully in the past to treat GAE in combination with the drugs listed, pentamidine is associated with adverse effects including nephrotoxicity, leukopenia, elevated liver enzymes, and hypoglycemia. Additionally, pentamidine does not cross the normal, intact blood-brain barrier well.
10. Miltefosine is not approved for any indication in the US. Case reports and *in vitro* data suggest it may have some anti-amebic activity (AC Aichelburg et al, Emerg Infect Dis 2008; 14:1743; DY Martinez et al, Infect Dis Soc Amer 2010; 51:e7; FL Schuster et al, J Eukaryot Microbiol 2006; 53:121). Miltefosine *(Impavido)* is manufactured in 10- or 50-mg capsules by Paladin (Canada) and is available in the US from the CDC for treatment of infections with free-living amebae. The drug is contraindicated in breastfeeding and pregnant women; a negative pregnancy test before drug initiation and effective contraception during and for 4 months after treatment is recommended (HW Murray et al, Lancet 2005; 366:1561).
11. LC Cary et al, Pediatrics 2010; 125:e699.
12. TR Deetz et al, Clin Infect Dis 2003;3 7:1304.
13. DY Martinez et al, Clin Infect Dis 2010; 51:e7.
14. LD Orozco et al, J Clin Neurosci 2011; 18:1118.
15. FG Bravo et al, Curr Opin Infect Dis 2011; 24:112.
16. JS Doyle et al, J Neurosurgery 2011;114: 458.

ANCYLOSTOMA caninum (Eosinophilic enterocolitis)

		Adult dosage	Pediatric dosage
Drug of choice:	Albendazole[1,2]	400 mg PO once	400 mg PO once
OR	Mebendazole	100 mg PO bid x 3d	100 mg PO bid x 3d
OR	Endoscopic removal		

1. Not FDA-approved for this indication.
2. Albendazole must be taken with food; a fatty meal increases oral bioavailability.

ANCYCLOSTOMA duodenale

See HOOKWORM

ANGIOSTRONGYLIASIS *(Angiostrongylus cantonensis, Angiostrongylus costaricensis)*

Drug of choice: *A. cantonensis* causes predominantly neurotropic disease.[1] *A. costaricensis* causes gastrointestinal disease. Most patients infected with either species have a self-limited course and recover completely. Analgesics, corticosteroids and periodic removal of CSF can relieve symptoms from increased intracranial pressure.[2] Treatment of *A. cantonensis* is controversial and varies across endemic areas.[3] No antihelminthic drug is proven to be effective and some patients have worsened with therapy. Mebendazole or albendazole each with or without a corticosteroid appear to shorten the course of infection.[4] Ocular angiostrongyliasis is managed by early and complete surgical removal of larva.[5]

1. QP Wang et al, Lancet Infect Dis 2008; 8:621.
2. L Ramirez-Avila et al, Clin Infect Dis 2009; 48:322.
3. Z Diao et al, Emerg Infect Dis 2011; 17:e1.
4. K Sawanyawisuth and K Sawanyawisuth, Trans R Soc Trop Med Hyg 2008; 102:990; V Chotmongkol et al, Am J Trop Med Hyg 2009; 81:443.
5. Z Diao et al, Trop Doctor 2011; 41:76.

ANISAKIASIS (*Anisakis* spp.)

	Drug	Adult dosage	Pediatric dosage
Treatment of choice:[1]	Surgical or endoscopic removal		

1. Gastric anisakiasis can usually be diagnosed and treated by endoscopic removal of the worm (NS Hochberg and DH Hamer, Clin Infect Dis 2010; 51:806). Enteric anisakiasis is more difficult to diagnose; capsule or double balloon endoscopy has been used (H Yasunaga et al, Am J Trop Med Hyg 2010; 83:104; K Nakaji, Intern Med 2009; 48:573). Disease can be managed without worm removal as the worms eventually die. Surgery may be needed in the event of intestinal obstruction or peritonitis (A Repiso Ortega et al, Gastroenterol Hepatol 2003; 26:341). Successful treatment of anisakiasis with albendazole 400 mg PO bid x 3-5d has been reported, but diagnosis was presumptive (DA Moore et al, Lancet 2002; 360:54; E Pacios et al, Clin Infect Dis 2005; 41:1825).

ASCARIASIS (*Ascaris lumbricoides,* roundworm)

	Drug	Adult dosage	Pediatric dosage
Drug of choice:[1]	Albendazole[2,3]	400 mg PO once	400 mg PO once
OR	Mebendazole	100 mg bid PO x 3d or 500 mg once	100 mg PO bid x 3d or 500 mg once
OR	Ivermectin[2,4]	150-200 mcg/kg PO once	150-200 mcg/kg PO once

1. Nitazoxanide may be effective against a variety of protozoan and helminth infections (DA Bobak, Curr Infect Dis Rep 2006; 8:91; E Diaz et al, Am J Trop Med Hyg 2003; 68:384). It is effective against mild to moderate amebiasis, 500 mg bid x 3d (JF Rossignol et al, Trans R Soc Trop Med Hyg 2007; 101:1025; AE Escobedo et al, Arch Dis Child 2009; 94:478). It is FDA-approved only for treatment of diarrhea caused by *Giardia* or *Cryptosporidium* (Med Lett Drugs Ther 2003; 45:29). Nitazoxanide is available in 500-mg tablets and an oral suspension; it should be taken with food.
2. Not FDA-approved for this indication.
3. Albendazole must be taken with food; a fatty meal increases oral bioavailability.
4. P Gonzalez et al, Curr Pharm Biotechnol 2012; 13:1103. Safety of ivermectin in young children (<15 kg) and pregnant women remains to be established; animal studies have shown adverse effects on the fetus (IM el-Ashmawy et al, Res Vet Sci 2011; 90:116). Taking ivermectin with a meal increases its bioavailability (CA Guzzo et al, J Clin Pharmacol 2002; 42:1122).

BABESIOSIS

	Drug	Adult dosage	Pediatric dosage
Drug of choice:[1]	Atovaquone[2,3]	750 mg PO bid x 7-10d	40 mg/kg/d PO in 2 doses x 7-10d
	plus azithromycin[2]	500-1000 mg PO on d1, then 250-500 mg PO on d2-10	10 mg/kg (max 500 mg/dose) PO on d1, then 5 mg/kg/d (max 250 mg dose) PO on d2-10
OR	Clindamycin[2,4]	300-600 mg IV qid or 600 mg PO tid x 7-10d	20-40 mg/kg/d (max 600 mg/dose) IV or PO in 3 or 4 doses x 7-10d
	plus quinine[2,5]	650 mg PO tid or qid x 7-10d	24 mg/kg/d (max 600 mg/dose) PO in 3 doses x 7-10d

1. *Babesia microti* is the most common cause of human babesiosis in the US (E Vannier and PJ Krause, N Engl J Med 2012; 366:2397), but disease caused by *B. duncani* or *B. divergens*-like organisms also has been documented (DH Persing et al, N Engl J Med 1995; 332:298; B Herwaldt et al, Ann Intern Med 1996; 124:643). In Europe, most cases have been attributed to *B. divergens* whereas a few have been caused by *B. venatorum* or *B. microti* (BL Herwaldt et al, Emerg Infect Dis 2003; 9:942; KP Hunfeld et al, Int J Parasitol 2008; 38:1219). *B. microti*-like organisms have been identified as etiologic agents in cases reported from Japan and Taiwan. Concurrent babesiosis, Lyme disease and/or human granulocytic anaplasmosis may occur (C Thompson et al, Clin Infect Dis 2001; 33:676).

   Symptoms of *B. microti* infection typically are mild to moderate and are treated with atovaquone plus azithromycin (PJ Krause et al, N Engl J Med 2000; 343:1454). Clindamycin plus quinine is recommended for severe symptoms with *B. microti* infection and for all *B. divergens* infections (GP Wormser et al, Clin Infect Dis 2006; 43:1089; E Vannier and PJ Krause, N Engl J Med 2012; 366:2397). Clindamycin plus quinine is also the treatment of choice for infections caused by *B. duncani*, *B. divergens*-like organisms or *B. venatorum*. Exchange tranfusion should be considered for severely ill patients and those with high (>10%) parasitemia or pulmonary, renal or hepatic compromise when infection is caused by *B. microti* and is recommended for cases of *B. divergens* infection. Highly immunosuppressed patients should be treated for a minimum of 6 weeks and at least 2 weeks past the last positive smear (PJ Krause et al, Clin Infect Dis 2008; 46:370). High doses of azithromycin (600-1000 mg) have been used in combination with atovaquone for the treatment of immunocompromised patients (LM Weiss et al, N Engl J Med 2001; 344:773). Resistance to atovaquone plus azithromycin has been reported in immunocompromised patients treated with a single subcurative course of this regimen (GP Wormser et al, Clin Infect Dis 2010; 50:381).
2. Not FDA-approved for this indication.
3. Atovaquone is available in an oral suspension that should be taken with a meal to increase absorption.
4. Oral clindamycin should be taken with a full glass of water to minimize esophageal ulceration.
5. Quinine should be taken with or after a meal to decrease gastrointestinal adverse effects.

BALAMUTHIA mandrillaris

See AMEBIC MENINGOENCEPHALITIS, PRIMARY

BALANTIDIASIS *(Balantidium coli)*

	Drug	Adult dosage	Pediatric dosage
Drug of choice:	Tetracycline[1,2]	500 mg PO qid x 10d	40 mg/kg/d (max 2 g) PO in 4 doses x 10d
Alternative:	Metronidazole[1]	500-750 mg PO tid x 5d	35-50 mg/kg/d PO in 3 doses x 5d
OR	Iodoquinol[1,3]	650 mg PO tid x 20d	30-40 mg/kg/d (max 2 g) PO in 3 doses x 20d

1. Not FDA-approved for this indication.
2. Use of tetracyclines is contraindicated in pregnancy and in children <8 years old. Tetracycline should be taken 1 hour before or 2 hours after meals and/or dairy products.
3. Iodoquinol should be taken after meals.

BAYLISASCARIASIS *(Baylisascaris procyonis)*

	Drug	Adult dosage	Pediatric dosage
Drug of choice:	The combination of albendazole 37 mg/kg/d PO and high-dose steroids has been used successfully.[1,2] Albendazole 25 mg/kg/d PO x 20d started as soon as possible (up to 3d after possible infection) might prevent clinical disease and is recommended for children with known exposure (ingestion of raccoon stool or contaminated soil).[3] Mebendazole, levamisole or ivermectin could be tried if albendazole is not available. Ocular baylisascariasis has been treated successfully using laser photocoagulation therapy to destroy the intraretinal larvae.[4]		

1. JM Peters et al, Pediatrics 2012; 129:e806.
2. S Haider, Emerg Infect Dis 2012; 18:347.
3. WJ Murray and KR Kazacos, Clin Infect Dis 2004; 39:1484.
4. CA Garcia et al, Eye (Lond) 2004; 18:624.

BLASTOCYSTIS spp.

	Drug	Adult dosage	Pediatric dosage
Drug of choice:	Clinical significance of these organisms is controversial.[1] Treatment options include metronidazole 750 mg PO tid x 10d, trimethoprim/sulfamethoxazole 1 DS tab PO bid x 7d or iodoquinol 650 mg PO tid x 20d.[2] Metronidazole resistance may be common in some areas.[3] Nitazoxanide has been effective in clearing organisms and improving symptoms.[4]		

1. P Poirier et al, PLoS Pathogens 2012; 8:e1002545.
2. KS Tan, Clin Microbiol Rev 2008; 21:639.
3. J Yakoob et al, Br J Biomed Sci 2004; 61:75.
4. E Diaz et al, Am J Trop Med Hyg 2003; 68:384; JF Rossignol, Clin Gastroenterol Hepatol 2005; 3:987.

CAPILLARIASIS *(Capillaria philippinensis)*

	Drug	Adult dosage	Pediatric dosage
Drug of choice:	Mebendazole[1]	200 mg PO bid x 20d	200 mg PO bid x 20d
Alternative:	Albendazole[1,2]	400 mg PO daily x 10d	400 mg PO daily x 10d

1. Not FDA-approved for this indication.
2. Albendazole must be taken with food; a fatty meal increases oral bioavailability.

CHAGAS' DISEASE

See TRYPANOSOMIASIS

CLONORCHIS sinensis

See FLUKE infection

CRYPTOSPORIDIOSIS *(Cryptosporidium)*

	Drug	Adult dosage	Pediatric dosage
Immunocompetent			
Drug of choice:	Nitazoxanide[1]	500 mg PO bid x 3d	1-3yrs: 100 mg PO bid x 3d 4-11yrs: 200 mg PO bid x 3d >12yrs: 500 mg PO bid x 3d
Immunocompromised			
Drug of choice:	No drug has proven efficacy in cryptosporidiosis in immunosuppressed patients.[2] For HIV-infected patients, potent antiretroviral therapy (ART) is the mainstay of treatment. Nitazoxanide (treatment duration of 5-21 days),[3] paromomycin, or a combination of paromomycin and azithromycin may be tried to decrease diarrhea and recalcitrant malabsorption of antimicrobial drugs, which can occur with chronic cryptosporidiosis.[4]		

1. Nitazoxanide may be effective against a variety of protozoan and helminth infections (DA Bobak, Curr Infect Dis Rep 2006; 8:91; E Diaz et al, Am J Trop Med Hyg 2003; 68:384). It is effective against mild to moderate amebiasis, 500 mg bid x 3d (JF Rossignol et al, Trans R Soc Trop Med Hyg 2007; 101:1025; AA Escobedo et al, Arch Dis Child 2009; 94:478), but perhaps less so than metronidazole (S Becker et al, Am J Trop Med Hyg 2011; 84:581). Nitazoxanide is FDA-approved only for treatment of diarrhea caused by *Giardia* or *Cryptosporidium* (Med Lett Drugs Ther 2003; 45:29). It is available in 500-mg tablets and an oral suspension and should be taken with food.
2. GJ Leitch and Q He, J Biomed Res 2012; 25:1.
3. I Krause et al, Pediatr Infect Dis J 2012; 31:1135.
4. B Pantenburg et al, Expert Rev Anti Infect Ther 2009; 7:385.

CUTANEOUS LARVA MIGRANS (creeping eruption, dog and cat hookworm)

	Drug	Adult dosage	Pediatric dosage
Drug of choice:[1]	Albendazole[2,3]	400 mg PO daily x 3d	400 mg PO daily x 3d
OR	Ivermectin[2,4]	200 mcg/kg PO daily x 1-2d	200 mcg/kg PO daily x 1-2d

1. J Heukelbach and H Feldmeier, Lancet Infect Dis 2008; 8:302; DD Bowman et al, Trends Parasitol 2012; 26:162.
2. Not FDA-approved for this indication.
3. Albendazole must be taken with food; a fatty meal increases oral bioavailability.
4. P Gonzalez et al, Curr Pharm Biotechnol 2012; 13:1103. Safety of ivermectin in young children (<15 kg) and pregnant women remains to be established; animal studies have shown adverse effects on the fetus (IM el-Ashmawy et al, Res Vet Sci 2011; 90:116). Taking ivermectin with a meal increases its bioavailability (CA Guzzo et al, J Clin Pharmacol 2002; 42:1122).

CYCLOSPORIASIS *(Cyclospora cayetanensis)*

	Drug	Adult dosage	Pediatric dosage
Drug of choice:[1]	Trimethoprim/ sulfamethoxazole[2]	TMP 160 mg/SMX 800 mg (1 DS tab) PO bid x 7-10d	TMP 10 mg/kg/SMX 50 mg/kg/d PO in 2 doses x 7-10d
Alternative:	Ciprofloxacin[2]	500 mg PO bid x 7d	–

1. YR Ortega and R Sanchez, Clin Microbiol Rev 2010; 23:218. In one study of HIV-infected patients with *Cyclospora* infection, ciprofloxacin treatment led to resolution in 87% of patients compared to 100% with TMP/SMX (RI Verdier et al, Ann Intern Med 2000; 132:885). HIV-infected patients may need higher dosage and long-term maintenance. Nitazoxanide (see also footnote 3) has also been used in a few patients, some of whom were sulfa-allergic (SM Zimmer et al, Clin Infect Dis 2007; 44:466; E Diaz et al, Am J Trop Med Hyg 2003; 68:384).
2. Not FDA-approved for this indication.
3. Nitazoxanide may be effective against a variety of protozoan and helminth infections (DA Bobak, Curr Infect Dis Rep 2006; 8:91; E Diaz et al, Am J Trop Med Hyg 2003; 68:384). It is effective against mild to moderate amebiasis, 500 mg bid x 3d (JF Rossignol et al, Trans R Soc Trop Med Hyg 2007; 101:1025; AA Escobedo et al, Arch Dis Child 2009; 94:478), but perhaps less so than metronidazole (S Becker et al, Am J Trop Hyg 2011; 84:581). Nitazoxanide is FDA-approved only for treatment of diarrhea caused by *Giardia* or *Cryptosporidium* (Med Lett Drugs Ther 2003; 45:29). It is available in 500-mg tablets and an oral suspension and should be taken with food.

CYSTICERCOSIS

See TAPEWORM infection

CYSTOISOSPORIASIS (*Cystoisospora belli,* formerly known as *Isospora*)

	Drug	Adult dosage	Pediatric dosage
Drug of choice:[1]	Trimethoprim/ sulfamethoxazole[2]	TMP 160 mg/SMX 800 mg (1 DS tab) PO bid x 10d	TMP 10 mg/kg/d/SMX 50 mg/kg/d PO in 2 doses x 10d

1. *Isospora belli* has been renamed and included in the *Cystoisospora* genus. Usually a self-limited illness in immunocompetent patients. Immunosuppressed patients may need higher doses and longer duration (TMP/SMX qid for up to 3 to 4 weeks (Morbid Mortal Wkly Rep 2009; 58 RR4:1). They may also require secondary prophylaxis (TMP/SMX DS tiw). In sulfa-allergic patients, pyrimethamine 50-75 mg daily in divided doses (plus leucovorin 10-25 mg/d) has been effective (LM Weiss et al, Ann Intern Med 1988; 109:474).
2. Not FDA-approved for this indication.

DIENTAMOEBA fragilis infection[1]

	Drug	Adult dosage	Pediatric dosage
Drug of choice:[2]	Paromomycin[4,5]	25-35 mg/kg/d PO in 3 doses x 7d	25-35 mg/kg/d PO in 3 doses x 7d
OR	Iodoquinol[3,4]	650 mg PO tid x 20d	30-40 mg/kg/d (max 2g) PO in 3 doses x 20d
OR	Metronidazole[4]	500-750 mg PO tid x 10d	35-50 mg/kg/d PO in 3 doses x 10d

1. D Stark et al, Am J Trop Med Hyg 2010; 82:614; O Vandenberg et al, Pediatr Infect Dis J 2007; 26:88; JL Barratt et al, Parasitology 2011; 138:557.
2. In one study, single-dose ornidazole, a nitroimidazole similar to metronidazole that is available in Europe, was effective and better tolerated than 5 days of metronidazole (O Kurt, Clin Microbiol Infect 2008; 14:601).
3. Iodoquinol should be taken after meals.
4. Not FDA-approved for this indication.
5. Paromomycin should be taken with a meal.

DIPHYLLOBOTHRIUM latum

See TAPEWORM infection

DRACUNCULUS medinensis (guinea worm) infection

	Drug	Adult dosage	Pediatric dosage
Drug of choice:	No drug is curative against *Dracunculus*. A program for monitoring local sources of drinking water to eliminate transmission has dramatically decreased the number of cases worldwide. The treatment of choice is slow extraction of worm combined with wound care and pain management.[1]		

1. MMWR Morbid Mortal Wkly Rep 2011; 60:1450.

ECHINOCOCCUS

See TAPEWORM infection

ENTAMOEBA histolytica

See AMEBIASIS infection

ENTEROBIUS vermicularis **(pinworm) infection**

	Drug	Adult dosage	Pediatric dosage
Drug of choice:[1]	Albendazole[2,3]	400 mg PO once; repeat in 2wks	400 mg PO once; repeat in 2wks
OR	Mebendazole	100 mg PO once; repeat in 2wks	100 mg PO once; repeat in 2wks
OR	Pyrantel pamoate[4]	11 mg/kg base PO once (max 1 g); repeat in 2wks	11 mg/kg base PO once (max 1 g); repeat in 2wks

1. Since family members are usually infected, treatment of the entire household is recommended; retreatment after 14-21d may be needed.
2. Not FDA-approved for this indication.
3. Albendazole must be taken with food; a fatty meal increases oral bioavailability.
4. Available without a prescription. Pyrantel pamoate suspension can be mixed with milk or fruit juice.

FASCIOLA hepatica

See FLUKE infection

FILARIASIS[1,2]

	Drug	Adult dosage	Pediatric dosage
Wuchereria bancrofti, Brugia malayi, Brugia timori			
Drug of choice:[3]	Diethylcarbamazine[4,5]	6 mg/kg/d PO in 3 doses x 1 or 12d[6]	6 mg/kg/d PO in 3 doses x 1 or 12d[6]
Loa loa			
Drug of choice:[7]	Diethylcarbamazine[4,5]	9 mg/kg/d PO in 3 doses x 21d[6]	9 mg/kg/d PO in 3 doses x 21d[6]
Mansonella ozzardi			
Drug of choice:	See footnote 8		
Mansonella perstans			
Drug of choice:	See footnote 9		
Mansonella streptocerca			
Drug of choice:[10]	Diethylcarbamazine[4,5]	6 mg/kg/d PO in 3 doses x 12d[6]	6 mg/kg/d PO in 3 doses x 12d[6]
OR	Ivermectin[5,11]	150 mcg/kg PO once	150 mcg/kg PO once
Tropical Pulmonary Eosinophilia (TPE)[12]			
Drug of choice:	Diethylcarbamazine[4,5]	6 mg/kg/d in 3 doses x 12-21d[6]	6 mg/kg/d in 3 doses x 12-21d[6]
Onchocerca volvulus (River blindness)			
Drug of choice:	Ivermectin[11,13]	150 mcg/kg PO once, repeated every 6-12 mos until asymptomatic	150 mcg/kg PO once, repeated every 6-12 mos until asymptomatic

1. Antihistamines or corticosteroids may be required to decrease allergic reactions to components of disintegrating microfilariae that result from treatment, especially in infection caused by *Loa loa*.
2. Endosymbiotic *Wolbachia* bacteria, which are present in most human filariae except *Loa loa*, are essential to filarial growth, development, embryogenesis and survival and represent an additional target for therapy. Doxycycline 100 or 200 mg/d PO x 6-8 wks in lymphatic filariasis, onchocerciasis, and *Mansonella perstans* has resulted in substantial loss of *Wolbachia* and decrease in both micro- and macrofilariae (MJ Bockarie et al, Expert Rev Anti Infect Ther 2009; 7:595; A Hoerauf, Curr Opin Infect Dis 2008; 21:673; YI Coulibaly et al, N Engl J Med 2009; 361:1448). Use of tetracyclines is contraindicated in pregnancy and in children <8 yrs old.

3. Most symptoms are caused by the adult worm. A single-dose combination of albendazole (400 mg PO) with either ivermectin (200 mcg/kg PO) or diethylcarbamazine (6 mg/kg PO) is effective for reduction or suppression of *W. bancrofti* microfilaria; none of these drug combinations kills all the adult worms (MJ Taylor et al, Lancet 2010; 376:1175).
4. Diethylcarbamazine is available from the CDC [(407) 718-4745; email: parasites@cdc.gov].
5. Not FDA-approved for this indication.
6. Multi-dose regimens have been shown to provide more rapid reduction in microfilaria than single-dose diethylcarbamazine, but microfilaria levels are similar 6-12 months after treatment (LD Andrade et al, Trans R Soc Trop Med Hyg 1995; 89:319; PE Simonsen et al, Am J Trop Med Hyg 1995; 53:267). A single dose of 6 mg/kg is used in endemic areas for mass treatment, but there are no studies directly comparing the efficacy of the single-dose regimen to a 12-day course. One review concluded that the 12-day regimen did not have a higher macrofilaricidal effect than single dose (A Hoerauf, Curr Opin Infect Dis 2008; 21: 673; J Figueredo-Silva et al, Trans R Soc Trop Med Hyg 1996; 90:192; J Noroes et al, Trans R Soc Trop Med Hyg 1997; 91:78). For patients with microfilaria in the blood, some Medical Letter consultants recommend starting with a lower dosage and scaling up: d1: 50 mg; d2: 50 mg tid; d3: 100 mg tid; d4-14: 6 mg/kg/d in 3 doses (for *Loa loa* d4-14: 9 mg/kg/d in 3 doses). Diethylcarbamazine should not be used for treatment of *Onchocerca volvulus* due to the risk of increased ocular side effects (including blindness) associated with rapid killing of the worms. It should be used cautiously in geographic regions where *O. volvulus* coexists with other filariae. See also footnote 13.
7. M Bossinesq, J Travel Med 2012; 19:140. In heavy infections with *Loa loa*, rapid killing of microfilariae can provoke encephalopathy. Apheresis has been reported to be effective in lowering microfilarial counts in patients heavily infected with *Loa loa* (EA Ottesen, Infect Dis Clin North Am 1993; 7:619). Albendazole may be useful for treatment of loiasis when diethylcarbamazine is ineffective or cannot be used, but repeated courses may be necessary (AD Klion et al, Clin Infect Dis 1999; 29:680; TE Tabi et al, Am J Trop Med Hyg 2004; 71:211). Ivermectin has also been used to reduce microfilaremia, but albendazole is preferred because of its slower onset of action and lower risk of precipitating encephalopathy (AD Klion et al, J Infect Dis 1993; 168:202; M Kombila et al, Am J Trop Med Hyg 1998; 58:458). Diethylcarbamazine, 300 mg PO once/wk, has been recommended for prevention of loiasis (TB Nutman et al, N Engl J Med 1988; 319:752).
8. Diethylcarbamazine has no effect. A single dose of ivermectin 200 mcg/kg PO reduces microfilaria densities and provides both short- and long-term reductions in *M. ozzardi* microfilaremia (AA Gonzalez et al, W Indian Med J 1999; 48:231). These parasites have been shown to contain *Wolbachia* which suggests doxycycline might be effective. See also footnote 2.
9. Diethylcarbamazine, melbendazole and ivermectin have not been found to be effective against *M. perstans*. Doxycycline is the drug of choice for disease acquired in West Africa (YI Coulibaly et al, N Engl J Med 2009; 361:1448). Strains from Uganda appear not to have *Wolbachia* (MP Grobusch et al, Parasitol Res 2003; 90:405). There is no effective therapy for patients with these strains or those who cannot take doxycycline (pregnant women, young children). See also footnote 2.

(continued)

FILARIASIS (continued)

10. Diethylcarbamazine is potentially curative due to activity against both adult worms and microfilariae. Geographic overlap with *Onchocerca volvulus* and inability of most labs to distinguish between the species limits its use (see also footnote 14). Ivermectin is active only against microfilariae and can lead to long-term suppression (P Fischer et al, J Infect Dis 1999; 180:1403). These parasites have been shown to contain *Wolbachia* which suggests doxycycline might be effective. See also footnote 2.
11. P Gonzalez et al, Curr Pharm Biotechnol 2012; 13:1103. Safety of ivermectin in young children (<15 kg) and pregnant women remains to be established; animal studies have shown adverse effects on the fetus (IM el-Ashmawy et al, Res Vet Sci 2011; 90:116). Taking ivermectin with a meal increases its bioavailability (CA Guzzo et al, J Clin Pharmacol 2002; 42:1122).
12. VK Vijayan, Curr Opin Pulm Med 2007; 13:428. Relapses occur and can be treated with a repeated course of diethylcarbamazine.
13. Diethylcarbamazine should not be used for treatment of this disease because rapid killing of the worms can lead to blindness. Periodic treatment with ivermectin (every 3-12 months), 150 mcg/kg PO, can prevent blindness due to ocular onchocerciasis (DN Udall, Clin Infect Dis 2007; 44:53). Skin reactions after ivermectin treatment are often reported in persons with high microfilarial skin densities. Ivermectin has been inadvertently given to pregnant women during mass treatment programs; the rates of congenital abnormalities were similar in treated and untreated women. Because of the high risk of blindness from onchocerciasis, the use of ivermectin after the first trimester is considered acceptable according to the WHO. Addition of 6-8 weeks of doxycycline to ivermectin is increasingly common. Doxycycline (100 mg/day PO for 6 weeks), alone or followed by a single 150 mcg/kg PO dose of ivermectin, resulted in long-term amicrofilaridermia and elimination of *Wolbachia* species (A Hoerauf et al, Lancet 2001; 357:1415; A Hoerauf et al, Parasitol Res 2009; 104:437).

FLUKE, hermaphroditic, infection

	Drug	Adult dosage	Pediatric dosage
Clonorchis sinensis (Chinese liver fluke)[1]			
Drug of choice:	Praziquantel[2]	75 mg/kg/d PO in 3 doses x 1-2d	75 mg/kg/d PO in 3 doses x 1-2d
OR	Albendazole[3,4]	10 mg/kg/d PO x 7d	10 mg/kg/d PO x 7d
Fasciola hepatica (sheep liver fluke)[1]			
Drug of choice:[5]	Triclabendazole[7]*	10 mg/kg PO once or twice	10 mg/kg PO once or twice
Alternative:	Bithionol*	30-50 mg/kg on alternate days x 10-15 doses	30-50 mg/kg on alternate days x 10-15 doses
OR	Nitazoxanide[3,6]	500 mg PO bid x 7d	1-3yrs: 100 mg PO bid x 7d 4-11yrs: 200 mg PO bid x 7d >12yrs: 500 mg PO bid x 7d
Fasciolopsis buski, Heterophyes heterophyes, Metagonimus yokogawai (intestinal flukes)			
Drug of choice:	Praziquantel[2,3]	75 mg/kg/d PO in 3 doses x 1d	75 mg/kg/d PO in 3 doses x 1d
Metorchis conjunctus (North American liver fluke)			
Drug of choice:	Praziquantel[2,3]	75 mg/kg/d PO in 3 doses x 1d	75 mg/kg/d PO in 3 doses x 1d
Nanophyetus salmincola			
Drug of choice:	Praziquantel[2,3]	60 mg/kg/d PO in 3 doses x 1d	60 mg/kg/d PO in 3 doses x 1d
Opisthorchis viverrini (Southeast Asian liver fluke)[1]			
Drug of choice:	Praziquantel[2]	75 mg/kg/d PO in 3 doses x 2d	75 mg/kg/d PO in 3 doses x 2d
OR	Albendazole[3,4]	10 mg/kg/d PO x 7d	10 mg/kg/d PO x 7d
Paragonimiasis (P. westermani, P. miyazaki, P. skrjabini, P. hueitungensis, P. heterotrema, P. utcerobilaterus, P. africanus, P. mexicanus, P. kellicotti) (lung fluke)			
Drug of choice:	Praziquantel[2,3]	75 mg/kg/d PO in 3 doses x 2d	75 mg/kg/d PO in 3 doses x 2d
Alternative:	Triclabendazole[7]*	10 mg/kg PO once or twice	10 mg/kg PO once or twice
	Bithionol*	30-50 mg/kg on alternate days x 10-15 doses	30-50 mg/kg on alternate days x 10-15 doses

(continued)

FLUKE, hermaphroditic, infection (continued)

* Availability problems. See table of manufacturers on pages 83–86.

1. LA Marcos, Curr Opin Infect Dis 2008; 21:523; ST Hong and Y Fang, Parasitol Int 2012; 61:17; J Keiser et al, Curr Opin Infect Dis 2010; 25:513.
2. Praziquantel should be taken with liquids during a meal.
3. Not FDA-approved for this indication.
4. Albendazole must be taken with food; a fatty meal increases oral bioavailability.
5. Unlike infections with other flukes, *Fasciola hepatica* infections may not respond to praziquantel. Triclabendazole (*Egaten* - Novartis) appears to be safe and effective, but data are limited (J Keiser et al, Expert Opin Investig Drugs 2005; 14:1513). It is available from Victoria Pharmacy, Zurich, Switzerland (www.pharmaworld.com; 011-4143-344-60-60) and should be given with food for better absorption. Nitazoxanide also appears to have efficacy in treating fascioliasis in adults and in children (L Favennec et al, Aliment Pharmacol Ther 2003; 17:265; JF Rossignol et al, Trans R Soc Trop Med Hyg 1998; 92:103; SM Kabil et al, Curr Ther Res 2000; 61:339).
6. Nitazoxanide may be effective against a variety of protozoan and helminth infections (DA Bobak, Curr Infect Dis Rep 2006; 8:91; E Diaz et al, Am J Trop Med Hyg 2003; 68:384). It is effective against mild to moderate amebiasis, 500 mg bid x 3d (JF Rossignol et al, Trans R Soc Trop Med Hyg 2007; 101:1025; AE Escobedo et al, Arch Dis Child 2009; 94:478), but perhaps less so than metronidazole (S Becker et al, Am J Trop Med Hyg 2011; 84:581). Nitazoxanide is FDA-approved only for treatment of diarrhea caused by *Giardia* or *Cryptosporidium* (Med Lett Drugs Ther 2003; 45:29). Nitazoxanide is available in 500-mg tablets and an oral suspension and should be taken with food.
7. J Keiser et al, Expert Opin Investig Drugs 2005; 14:1513. See footnote 5 for availability.

GIARDIASIS *(Giardia duodenalis)*

	Drug	Adult dosage	Pediatric dosage
Drug of choice:	Tinidazole[1]	2 g PO once	≥3yrs: 50 mg/kg PO once (max 2 g)
OR	Metronidazole[2]	250 mg PO tid x 5-7d	15 mg/kg/d PO in 3 doses x 5-7d
OR	Nitazoxanide[3]	500 mg PO bid x 3d	1-3yrs: 100 mg PO bid x 3d 4-11yrs: 200 mg PO bid x 3d >12yrs: 500 mg PO bid x 3d
Alternative:[4]	Paromomycin[2,5,6]	25-35 mg/kg/d PO in 3 doses x 5-10d	25-35 mg/kg/d PO in 3 doses x 5-10d
OR	Furazolidone*	100 mg PO qid x 7-10d	6 mg/kg/d PO in 4 doses x 7-10d
OR	Quinacrine[7,8]*	100 mg PO tid x 5d	6 mg/kg/d PO in 3 doses x 5d (max 300 mg/d)

* Availability problems. See table of manufacturers on pages 83–86.

1. A nitroimidazole similar to metronidazole, tinidazole appears to be as effective as metronidazole and better tolerated (Med Lett Drugs Ther 2004; 46:70). It should be taken with food to minimize GI adverse effects. For children and patients unable to take tablets, a pharmacist can crush the tablets and mix them with cherry syrup (*Humco*, and others). The syrup suspension is good for 7 days at room temperature and must be shaken before use (HB Fung and TL Doan, Clin Ther 2005; 27:1859). Ornidazole, a similar drug, is also used outside the US.
2. Not FDA-approved for this indication.
3. Nitazoxanide may be effective against a variety of protozoan and helminth infections (DA Bobak, Curr Infect Dis Rep 2006; 8:91; E Diaz et al, Am J Trop Med Hyg 2003; 68:384). It is effective against mild to moderate amebiasis, 500 mg bid x 3d (JF Rossignol et al, Trans R Soc Trop Med Hyg 2007; 101:1025; AA Escobedo et al, Arch Dis Child 2009; 94:478), but perhaps less so than metronidazole (S Becker et al, Am J Trop Med Hyg 2011; 84:581. Nitazoxanide is FDA-approved only for treatment of diarrhea caused by *Giardia* or *Cryptosporidium* (Med Lett Drugs Ther 2003; 45:29). It is available in 500-mg tablets and an oral suspension and should be taken with food.

(continued)

GIARDIASIS (continued)

4. Additional option: albendazole (400 mg/d PO x 5d in adults and 10 mg/kg/d PO x 5d in children) (K Yereli et al, Clin Microbiol Infect 2004; 10:527; O Karabay et al, World J Gastroenterol 2004; 10:1215). Refractory disease: combination therapy with tinidazole or metronidazole plus paromomycin, furazolidine or quinacrine has been successful (TE Nash et al, Clin Infect Dis 2001; 33:22; R Lopez-Velez et al. Am J Trop Med Hyg 2010; 83:171). In one study, nitazoxanide was used successfully in high doses (1.5 g PO bid x 30d) to treat a case of *Giardia* resistant to metronidazole and albendazole (P Abboud et al, Clin Infect Dis 2001; 32:1792).
5. Paromomycin should be taken with a meal.
6. Poorly absorbed; may be useful for treatment of giardiasis in pregnancy.
7. Not available commercially. It may be obtained through compounding pharmacies such as Expert Compounding Pharmacy, 6744 Balboa Blvd, Lake Balboa, CA 91406 (800-247-9767) or Medical Center Pharmacy, New Haven, CT (203-688-7064). Other compounding pharmacies may be found through the National Association of Compounding Pharmacies (800-687-7850) or the Professional Compounding Centers of America (800-331-2498, www.pccarx.com).
8. Quinacrine should be taken with liquids after a meal.

GNATHOSTOMIASIS *(Gnathostoma spinigerum)*[1]

	Drug	Adult dosage	Pediatric dosage
Treatment of choice:	Albendazole[2,3]	400 mg PO bid x 21d	400 mg PO bid x 21d
OR	Ivermectin[2,4]	200 mcg/kg/d PO x 2d	200 mcg/kg/d PO x 2d
	either		
±	Surgical removal		

1. All patients should be treated with medication whether surgery is attempted or not. JS Herman and PL Chiodini, Clin Microbiol Rev 2009; 22:484; L Ramirez-Avila et al, Clin Infect Dis 2009; 48:322.
2. Not FDA-approved for this indication.
3. Albendazole must be taken with food; a fatty meal increases oral bioavailability.
4. P Gonzalez et al, Curr Pharm Biotechnol 2012; 13:1103. Safety of ivermectin in young children (<15 kg) and pregnant women remains to be established; animal studies have shown adverse effects on the fetus (IM el-Ashmawy et al, Res Vet Sci 2011; 90:116). Taking ivermectin with a meal increases its bioavailability (CA Guzzo et al, J Clin Pharmacol 2002; 42:1122).

GONGYLONEMIASIS (*Gongylonema* spp.)[1]

	Drug	Adult dosage	Pediatric dosage
Treatment of choice:	Surgical removal		
OR	Albendazole[2,3]	400 mg/d PO x 3d	400 mg/d PO x 3d

1. S Pasuralertsakul et al, Am Trop Med Parasitol 2008; 102:455; G Molavi et al, J Helminth 2006; 80:425.
2. Not FDA-approved for this indication.
3. Albendazole must be taken with food; a fatty meal increases oral bioavailability.

HOOKWORM infection *(Ancylostoma duodenale, Necator americanus)*

	Drug	Adult dosage	Pediatric dosage
Drug of choice:	Albendazole[1,2]	400 mg PO once	400 mg PO once
OR	Mebendazole	100 mg PO bid x 3d or 500 mg once	100 mg PO bid x 3d or 500 mg once
OR	Pyrantel pamoate[1,3]	11 mg/kg base (max 1g) PO daily x 3d	11 mg/kg base (max 1g) PO daily x 3d

1. Not FDA-approved for this indication.
2. Albendazole must be taken with food; a fatty meal increases oral bioavailability.
3. Available without a prescription. Pyrantel pamoate suspension can be mixed with milk or fruit juice.

HYDATID cyst

See TAPEWORM infection

HYMENOLEPIS nana

See TAPEWORM infection

ISOSPORA belli

See Cystoisospora

LEISHMANIASIS[1]

		Drug	Adult dosage	Pediatric dosage
Visceral[2,3]				
Drug of choice:		Liposomal amphotericin B	See footnote 4	See footnote 4
Alternative:		Sodium stibogluconate*	20 mg Sb/kg/d IV or IM x 28d	20 mg Sb/kg/d IV or IM x 28d
	OR	Meglumine antimonate*	20 mg Sb/kg/d IV or IM x 28d	20 mg Sb/kg/d IV or IM x 28d
	OR	Miltefosine[5,6]*	2.5 mg/kg/d PO (max 150 mg/d) x 28d	2.5 mg/kg/d PO (max 150 mg/d) x 28d
	OR	Amphotericin B[7]	1 mg/kg IV daily x 15-20d or every second day for 4-8 wks (total usually 15-20 mg/kg)	1 mg/kg IV daily x 15-20d or every second day for 4-8 wks (total usually 15-20 mg/kg)
	OR	Paromomycin[7,8]* sulfate	15 mg/kg/d IM x 21d	15 mg/kg/d IM x 21d
Cutaneous[1,2,9]				
Drugs of choice:		Sodium stibogluconate*	20 mg Sb/kg/d IV or IM x 20d	20 mg Sb/kg/d IV or IM x 20d
	OR	Meglumine antimonate*	20 mg Sb/kg/d IV or IM x 20d	20 mg Sb/kg/d IV or IM x 20d
	OR	Miltefosine[5,10]*	2.5 mg/kg/d PO (max 150 mg/d) x 28d	2.5 mg/kg/d PO (max 150 mg/d) x 28d
Alternative:[11]		Paromomycin[7,12]*	Topically 2x/d x 10-20d	Topically 2x/d x 10-20d
	OR	Pentamidine[7]	2-3 mg/kg IV or IM daily or every second day x 4-7 doses	2-3 mg/kg IV or IM daily or every second day x 4-7 doses

(continued)

LEISHMANIASIS (continued)

Mucosal[1,2,13]

		Drug	Adult dosage	Pediatric dosage
Drug of choice:		Sodium stibogluconate*	20 mg Sb/kg/d IV or IM x 28d	20 mg Sb/kg/d IV or IM x 28d
	OR	Meglumine antimonate*	20 mg Sb/kg/d IV or IM x 28d	20 mg Sb/kg/d IV or IM x 28d
	OR	Amphotericin B[7,14]	0.5-1 mg/kg IV daily or every second day for 4-8wks	0.5-1 mg/kg IV daily or every second day for 4-8wks
	OR	Miltefosine[5,15]*	2.5 mg/kg/d PO (max 150 mg/d) x 28d	2.5 mg/kg/d PO (max 150 mg/d) x 28d

* Availability problems. See table of manufacturers on pages 83–86.

1. HW Murray, Am J Trop Med Hyg 2012; 86:4346
2. Medical Letter reviewers recommend consultation with physicians experienced in management of this disease. To maximize effectiveness and minimize toxicity, the choice of drug, dosage and duration of therapy should be individualized based on the region of disease acquisition, likely infecting species, number, significance and location of lesions, and host factors such as immune status (HW Murray, Lancet 2005; 366:1561). Some of the listed drugs and regimens are effective only against certain *Leishmania* species/strains and only in certain areas of the world (S Sundar and J Chakravarty, Expert Opin Pharmacother 2013; 14:53).
3. Visceral infection is most commonly due to the Old World species *L. donovani* (kala-azar) and *L. infantum* (referred to as *L. chagasi* in the New World) (J van Griensven and E Diro, Infect Clin Dis Clin North Am 2012; 26:309).
4. Liposomal amphotericin B is the only lipid formulation of amphotericin B FDA approved for treatment of visceral leishmania, largely based on trials in patients infected with *L. infantum* (M Balasegaram et al, Expert Opin Emerg Drugs 2012; 17:493). It is the treatment of choice for visceral leishmaniasis in the US and Southern Europe and the treatment of choice for visceral disease in pregnancy. The total dose administered seems to be more important than the number of infusions or duration of therapy. The target dose for a non-immunocompromised host is 18-21 mg/kg over 5 days. Two doses of 10 mg/kg have been used successfully in children with disease acquired in the Mediterranean (V Syriopoulou et al, Clin Infect Dis 2003; 36:560). For visceral leishmaniasis acquired in the Indian subcontinent 10 mg/kg/day as a single dose or 5 days treatment with 3 mg/kg (total 15 mg/kg) has been effective (HW Murray et al, Lancet 2005; 366:1561; C Bern et al, Clin Infect Dis 2006; 43:917; S Sundar et al, N Engl J Med 2010; 362:504). The FDA-approved dosage regminen is 3 mg/kg/d IV on days 1-5, 14 and 21 and for immunocompromised patients is 4 mg/kg on days 1-5, 10, 17, 24, 31 and 38. The relapse rate in immunocompromised patients is high; maintenance therapy (secondary prevention) is generally given indicated, but there is no consensus on dosage and duration.

5. TP Dorlo et al, J Antimicrob Chemother 2012; 67:2576. Miltefosine *(Impavido)* is manufactured in 10- or 50-mg capsules by Paladin (Canada) and is available in the US from the manufacturer through an IND application from the FDA. The drug is contraindicated in breastfeeding and pregnant women; a negative pregnancy test before drug initiation and effective contraception during and for 4 months after treatment is recommended (HW Murray et al, Lancet 2005; 366:1561).
6. Miltefosine is effective for both antimony-sensitive and -resistant *L. donovani* (Indian).
7. Not FDA-approved for this indication.
8. Paromomycin IM has been effective against *Leishmania* in India and against visceral leishmaniasis in East Africa, although higher doses (20 mg/kg) or longer duration of therapy may be needed (AH Musa et al, PLoS Negl Trop Dis 2010; 4:e855; A Hailu et al, PLoS Negl Trop Dis 2010; 4:e709. There are insufficient data to support its use in pregnancy (S Sundar et al, N Engl J Med 2007; 356:2571; S Sundar and J Chakravarty, Expert Opin Investig Drugs 2008; 17:787). There is limited experience in paromomycin in South America or the Mediterranean where it has been tried as second-line combination therapy with sodium stibogluconate.
9. Cutaneous infection is most commonly due to the Old World species *L. major* and *L. tropica* and the New World species *L. mexicana, L. (Vianna) braziliensis, L. (V.) panamensis* and others.
10. PR Machado and G Penna, Curr Opin Infect Dis 2012; 25:141. Miltefosine has been effective in trials for treatment of cutaneous leishmaniasis due to *L.(V.) panamensis* in Bolivia and Colombia, and for *L.(V.) braziliensis* in Brazil but not for treatment of *L.(V.) braziliensis* or *L. mexicana* in Guatemala, suggesting geography as well as species affects efficacy (J Soto et al, Am J Trop Med Hyg 2008; 78:210, PR Machado et al, PLoS Negl Trop Dis 2010; 4:e912, J Soto et al, Clin Infect Dis 2004; 38:1266; LC Rubiano et al, J Infect Dis 2012; 205:684). It has also has been effective for treatment of *L. major* acquired in Afghanistan and Iran (M Mohebali et al, Acta Trop 2007; 103:33; PP van Thiel et al, Clin Infect Dis 50:80). For forms of disease that require long periods of treatment, such as diffuse cutaneous leishmaniasis and post kala-azar dermal leishmaniasis, miltefosine might be a useful treatment (JJ Berman, Expert Opin Drug Metab Toxicol 2008; 4:1209).

(continued)

LEISHMANIASIS (continued)

11. Azole drugs (fluconazole, ketoconazole, itraconazole) have been used to treat cutaneous disease, with plausible efficacy (JA Blum and CS Hatz, J Travel Med 2009; 16:123). For treatment of *L. major* cutaneous lesions, a study in Saudi Arabia found that oral fluconazole, 200 mg once/d x 6 wks appeared to modestly accelerate the healing process (AA Alrajhi et al, N Engl J Med 2002; 346:891). Fluconazole 8 mg/kg/d PO x 4-6 wks may have efficacy against *L. braziliensis* (AQ Sousa et al, Clin Infect Dis 2011; 53:693). Intralesional injections of sodium stibogluconate or topical paromomycinare also used for uncomplicated lesions when subsequent mucosal leshmaniasis is unlikely (J Soto et al, Clin Infect Dis 2013; 56:1255). Ketoconazole 600 mg/day PO x28-30 days has been effective against *L. major, L. panamenesis* and *L. mexicana.* Studies with liposomal amphotericin are limited; the FDA total approved dose of 21 mg/kg may be effective (G Wortmann et al, Am J Trop Hyg 2010; 83:1028). Thermotherapy may be an option for some cases of cutaneous *L. tropica* infection (R Reithinger et al, Clin Infect Dis 2005; 40:1148). A device that generates focused and controlled heating of the skin is being marketed (*ThermoMed* – ThermoSurgery Technologies Inc., Phoenix, AZ, 602-264-7300; www.thermosurgery.com). In a few studies, localized thermal heat was as effective as multiple doses of sodium stibogluconate or meglumine antimoniate for up to 18 months with less toxicity (N Safi et al, Mil Med 2012; 177:345; L Lopez et al, Trials 2012; 13:58; RA Bumb et al, Br J Dermatol 2013; Jan 8).
12. Topical paromomycin should be used only in geographic regions where cutaneous leishmaniasis species have low potential for mucosal spread. A formulation of 15% paromomycin/12% methylbenzethonium chloride *(Leshcutan)* in soft white paraffin for topical use has been reported to be partially effective against cutaneous leishmaniasis due to *L. major* in Israel and Tunesia and *L. mexicana* and *L. (V.) braziliensis* in Guatemala, where mucosal spread is very rare (BA Arana et al, Am J Trop Med Hyg 2001; 65:466; DH Kim et al, PLoS Negl Trop Dis 2009; 3:e381; A Ben Salah et al, N Engl J Med 2013; 368:524). The methylbenzethonium is irritating to the skin; lesions may worsen before they improve.
13. Mucosal infection (espundia) is most commonly due to New World species *L. (V.) braziliensis, L. (V.) panamensis,* or *L. (V.) guyanensis.*
14. Liposomal amphotericin 20-35 mg/kg divided in 3-5 doses may be active for mucosal disease (VS Amato et al, Am J Trop Med Hyg 2011; 85:818).
15. Miltefosine has been effective for mucosal leishmania due to *L.(V.) braziliensis* in Bolivia (J Soto et al, Clin Infect Dis 2007; 44:350; J Soto et al, Am J Trop Med Hyg 2009; 81:387).

LICE infestation (*Pediculus humanus, P. capitis, Phthirus pubis*)[1]

		Drug	Adult dosage	Pediatric dosage
Drug of choice:		Pyrethrins with piperonyl butoxide[2]	Topically, 2 x at least 7d apart	Topically, 2 x at least 7d apart
	OR	0.5% Ivermectin lotion[3]	Topically, once	Topically, once
	OR	0.9% Spinosad susp[4]	Topically, 2 x at least 7d apart	Topically, 2 x at least 7d apart
	OR	1% Permethrin[2]	Topically, 2 x at least 7d apart	Topically, 2 x at least 7d apart
	OR	5% Benzyl alcohol lotion[5]	Topically, 2 x at least 7d apart	Topically, 2 x at least 7d apart
	OR	0.5% Malathion[6]	Topically, 2 x at least 7d apart	Topically, 2 x at least 7d apart
Alternative:		Ivermectin[7,8,9]	200 or 400 mcg/kg PO	≥15 kg: 200 or 400 mcg/kg PO

1. Pediculocides should not be used for infestations of the eyelashes. Such infestations are treated with petrolatum ointment applied 2-4x/d x 8-10d. For pubic lice, treat with 1% permethrin, pyrethrins with piperonyl butoxide, or ivermectin.
2. Permethrin and pyrethrin are pediculocidal; retreatment in 7-10d is needed to eradicate the infestation. Some lice are resistant to pyrethrins and permethrin (TL Meinking et al, Arch Dermatol 2002; 138:220). Medical Letter consultants prefer pyrethrin products with a benzyl alcohol vehicle. Pyrethrins with piperonyl butoxide are recommended for use in children ≥2 years old; permethrin for children ≥2 months old.
3. Not ovicidal but lice that hatch from treated eggs die within 48 hours after hatching. Recommended for use in children ≥6 months old (Med Lett Drugs Ther 2012; 54:61; DM Pariser et al, N Engl J Med 2012; 367:1687).
4. Not ovicidal, but causes neuronal excitation in insects leading to paralysis and death. The formulation also includes benzyl alcohol, which is pediculocidal. Two applications 7 days apart are needed. Recommended for children ≥4 years old (Med Lett Drugs Ther 2011; 53:50).
5. Benzyl alcohol prevents lice from closing their respiratory spiracles and the lotion vehicle then obstructs their airway causing them to asphyxiate. It is not ovicidal. Two applications at least 7 days apart are needed. Recommended for use in children ≥6 months old. Resistance, which is a problem with other drugs, is unlikely to develop (Med Lett Drugs Ther 2009; 51:57).
6. Malathion is both ovicidal and pediculocidal; 2 applications at least 7 days apart are generally necessary to kill all lice and nits. Recommended for children ≥6 years old.
7. Not FDA-approved for this indication.

(continued)

LICE infestation (continued)

8. P Gonzalez et al, Curr Pharm Biotechnol 2012; 13:1103. Safety of ivermectin in young children (<15 kg) and pregnant women remains to be established; animal studies have shown adverse effects on the fetus (IM el-Ashmawy et al, Res Vet Sci 2011; 90:116). Taking ivermectin with a meal increases its bioavailability (CA Guzzo et al, J Clin Pharmacol 2002; 42:1122).
9. Ivermectin is pediculocidal, but not ovicidal; more than one dose is generally necessary to eradicate the infestation (KN Jones and JC English 3rd, Clin Infect Dis 2003; 36:1355). The number of doses and interval between doses has not been established; animal studies have shown adverse effects on the fetus (IM el-Ashmawy et al, Res Vet Sci 2011; 90:116). In one study of treatment of head lice, 2 doses of ivermectin (400 mcg/kg) 7 days apart were more effective than treatment with topical malathion (O Chosidow et al, N Engl J Med 2010; 362:896). In one study of treatment of body lice, a regimen of 3 doses of ivermectin (12 mg each) administered at 7-day intervals was effective (C Fouault et al, J Infect Dis 2006; 193:474).

LOA loa

See FILARIASIS

MALARIA, Treatment of *(Plasmodium falciparum,[1] P. vivax,[2] P. ovale, P. malariae[3] and P. knowlesi[4])*

		Drug	Adult dosage	Pediatric dosage
ORAL (Uncomplicated or mild infection)[5]				
***P. falciparum* or unidentified species[6] acquired in areas of chloroquine-resistant *P. falciparum*[1]**				
Drug of choice:		Atovaquone/ proguanil[7]	4 adult tabs PO once/d or 2 adult tabs PO bid[8] x 3d	<5kg: not indicated 5-8kg: 2 peds tabs PO once/d x 3d 9-10kg: 3 peds tabs PO once/d x 3d 11-20kg: 1 adult tab PO once/d x 3d 21-30kg: 2 adult tabs PO once/d x 3d 31-40kg: 3 adult tabs PO once/d x 3d >40kg: 4 adult tabs PO once/d x 3d[8]
	OR	Artemether/ lumefantrine[9,10]	6 doses over 3d (4 tabs/dose at 0, 8, 24, 36, 48 and 60 hours)	6 doses over 3d at same intervals as adults; 5-15kg: 1 tab/dose ≥15-25kg: 2 tabs/dose ≥25-35kg: 3 tabs/dose ≥35kg: 4 tabs/dose
	OR	Quinine sulfate	650 mg PO q8h x 3 **or** 7d[11]	30 mg/kg/d PO in 3 doses x 3 **or** 7d[11]
		plus doxycycline[12,13,14]	100 mg PO bid x 7d	4 mg/kg/d PO in 2 doses x 7d
		or plus tetracycline[12,13]	250 mg PO qid x 7d	25 mg/kg/d PO in 4 doses x 7d
		or plus clindamycin[12,15,16]	20 mg/kg/d PO in 3 doses x 7d[17]	20 mg/kg/d PO in 3 doses x 7d[17]
Alternative:		Mefloquine[18,19]	750 mg PO followed 12 hrs later by 500 mg	15 mg/kg PO followed 12 hrs later by 10 mg/kg

(continued)

MALARIA, Treatment of (continued)

	Drug	Adult dosage	Pediatric dosage
***P. vivax* acquired in areas of chloroquine-resistant *P. vivax*[2]**			
Drug of choice:	Quinine sulfate	650 mg PO q8h x 3 or 7d[11]	30 mg/kg/d PO in 3 doses x 3-7d[11]
	plus doxycycline[12,13,14]	100 mg PO bid x 7d	4 mg/kg/d PO in 2 doses x 7d
PLUS	primaquine phosphate[6,20]	30 mg base/d PO x 14d	0.5 mg/kg/d PO x 14d
Alternative[21]:	Atovaquone/ proguanil[7,22]	4 adult tabs PO once/d or 2 adult tabs bid[8] x 3d	<5kg: not indicated 5-8kg: 2 peds tabs PO once/d x 3d 9-10kg: 3 peds tabs PO once/d x 3d 11-20kg: 1 adult tab PO once/d x 3d 21-30kg: 2 adult tabs PO once/d x 3d 31-40kg: 3 adult tabs PO once/d x 3d >40kg: 4 adult tabs PO once/d x 3d[8]
	Mefloquine[18]	750 mg PO followed 12 hrs later by 500 mg	15 mg/kg PO followed 12 hrs later by 10 mg/kg
EITHER PLUS	primaquine phosphate[6,20]	30 mg base/d PO x 14d	0.5 mg/kg/d PO x 14d
***Plasmodium* species in areas without chloroquine resistance[1-4]**			
Drug of choice:	Chloroquine phosphate[6,23]	1 g (600 mg base) PO, then 500 mg (300 mg base) 6 hrs later, then 500 mg (300 mg base) at 24 and 48 hrs	10 mg base/kg (max 600 mg base) PO, then 5 mg base/kg 6 hrs later, then 5 mg base/kg at 24 and 48 hrs
OR	a regimen used for chloroquine-resistant species listed above		

PARENTERAL (severe infection)[5]

All *Plasmodium* species (Chloroquine-sensitive and resistant)

		Drug	Adult dosage	Pediatric dosage
Drug of choice:[6,24]		Quinidine gluconate[25]	10 mg/kg IV loading dose (max 600 mg) in normal saline over 1-2 hrs, followed by continuous infusion of 0.02 mg/kg/min until PO therapy can be started	10 mg/kg IV loading dose (max 600 mg) in normal saline over 1-2 hrs, followed by continuous infusion of 0.02 mg/kg/min until PO therapy can be started
	OR	Quinine dihydrochloride[25]*	20 mg/kg IV loading dose in 5% dextrose over 4 hrs, followed by 10 mg/kg over 2-4 hrs q8h (max 1800 mg/d) until PO therapy can be started	20 mg/kg IV loading dose in 5% dextrose over 4 hrs, followed by 10 mg/kg over 2-4 hrs q8h (max 1800 mg/d) until PO therapy can be started
	OR	Artesunate[9,26]*	2.4 mg/kg/dose IV x 3d at 0, 12, 24, 48 and 72 hrs	2.4 mg/kg/dose IV x 3d at 0, 12, 24, 48 and 72 hrs
		plus a second oral drug[26]		

* Availability problems. See table of manufacturers on pages 83-86.

1. Chloroquine-resistant *P. falciparum* occurs in all malarious areas except Central America (including Panama north and west of the Canal Zone), Mexico, Haiti, the Dominican Republic, Paraguay, northern Argentina, North and South Korea, Georgia, Armenia, most of rural China and some countries in the Middle East (chloroquine resistance has been reported in Yemen, Saudi Arabia and Iran). For treatment of multiple-drug-resistant *P. falciparum* in Southeast Asia, especially the greater Mekong region that includes Myanmar, Thailand, Cambodia and Vietnam, where mefloquine resistance is frequent, atovaquone/proguanil, quinine plus either doxycycline or clindamycin, or artemether/lumefantrine may be used.
2. Chloroquine-resistant *P. vivax* is a significant problem in Papua-New Guinea and Indonesia. There are also reports of resistance from Myanmar, Vietnam, Korea, India, the Solomon Islands, Vanuatu, Indonesia, Guyana, Brazil, Colombia and Peru (JK Baird, Clin Microbiol Rev 2009; 22:508).
3. Chloroquine-resistant *P. malariae* has been reported from Sumatra (JD Maguire et al, Lancet 2002; 360:58).

(continued)

MALARIA, Treatment of (continued)

4. Human infection with the simian species, *P. knowlesi* has been reported in Malaysia where it was initially misdiagnosed as *P. malariae*. Additional cases have been reported from Thailand, Myanmar, Singapore, the Thai-Burma border, and the Philippines (J Cox-Singh et al, Clin Infect Dis 2008; 46:165; MMWR 2009; 58:229). Treatment with the usual antimalarials, such as chloroquine and atovaquone/proguanil appears to be effective. In cases of severe infection, IV artesunate combined with oral artemether/lumefantrine or artesunate/mefloquine has been used successfully (BE Barber et al, Clin Infect Dis 2013; 56:383).
5. Uncomplicated or mild malaria may be treated with oral drugs. Severe malaria (e.g. impaired consciousness, parasitemia >5%, shock, etc.) should be treated with parenteral drugs (KS Griffin et al, JAMA 2007; 297:2264). Malaria breakthrough infection in a patient on prophylaxis should be treated with a different drug than the drug taken for prophylaxis.
6. Primaquine is given as part of primary treatment to prevent relapse after infection with *P. vivax* or *P. ovale*. Vivax malaria is a potentially more dangerous infection than previously thought (JK Baird et al, Microbiol Rev 2013; 26:36). See also footnote 20.
7. Atovaquone/proguanil is available as a fixed-dose combination tablet: adult tablets (*Malarone*; atovaquone 250 mg/proguanil 100 mg) and pediatric tablets (*Malarone Pediatric*; atovaquone 62.5 mg/proguanil 25 mg). To enhance absorption and reduce nausea and vomiting, it should be taken with food or a milky drink. Safety in pregnancy is unknown and use is generally not recommended, In a few small studies outcomes were normal in women treated with the combination in the 2nd and 3rd trimester (B Pasternak et al, Arch Intern Med 2011; 171:259; AK Boggild et al, Am J Trop Med Hyg 2007; 76:208). The drug should not be given to patients with severe renal impairment (creatinine clearance <30 mL/min). There have been isolated case reports of resistance in *P. falciparum* in Africa, but Medical Letter consultants do not believe there is a high risk for acquisition of *Malarone*-resistant disease (E Schwartz et al, Clin Infect Dis 2003; 37:450; A Farnert et al, BMJ 2003; 326:628; S Kuhn et al, Am J Trop Med Hyg 2005; 72:407; CT Happi et al, Malaria Journal 2006; 5:82).
8. Although approved for once-daily dosing, Medical Letter consultants usually divide the dose in two to decrease nausea and vomiting.
9. The artemisinin-derivatives, artemether and artesunate, are both frequently used globally in combination regimens to treat malaria. Both are available in oral, parenteral and rectal formulations, but manufacturing standards are not consistent (HA Karunajeewa et al, JAMA 2007; 297:2381; EA Ashley and NJ White, Curr Opin Infect Dis 2005; 18:531). Based on the few studies available, artemesinins have been relatively safe during pregnancy (I Adam et al, Am Trop Med Parisitol 2009; 103; 205), but some experts would not prescribe them in the 1st trimester (RL Clark, Reprod Toxicol 2009; 28:285; C Manyando et al, Malaria J 2012; 11:141).

10. Artemether/lumefantrine is available as a fixed-dose combination tablet (*Coartem* in the US and in countries with endemic malaria, *Riamet* in Europe and countries without endemic malaria); each tablet contains artemether 20 mg and lumefantrine 120 mg. It is FDA-approved for treatment of uncomplicated malaria and should not be used for severe infection or for prophylaxis. The tablets should be taken with fatty food (tablets may be crushed, mixed with 1-2 tsp water, and taken with milk). Artemether/lumefantrine should not be used in patients with cardiac arrhythmias, bradycardia, severe cardiac disease or QT prolongation. Concomitant use of drugs that prolong the QT interval or are metabolized by CYP2D6 is contraindicated (Med Lett Drugs Ther 2009; 51:75).
11. Available in the US in a 324-mg capsule; 2 capsules suffice for adult dosage. In Southeast Asia, relative resistance to quinine has increased and treatment should be continued for 7 days. For infections acquired elsewhere treatment can be given for 3d. Quinine should be taken with or after meals to decrease gastrointestinal adverse effects. It is generally considered safe in pregnancy.
12. Not FDA-approved for this indication.
13. Use of tetracyclines is contraindicated in pregnancy and in children <8 years old. Tetracycline should be taken 1 hour before or 2 hours after meals and/or dairy products.
14. Doxycycline should be taken with adequate water to avoid esophageal irritation. It can be taken with food to minimize gastrointestinal adverse effects.
15. Oral clindamycin should be taken with a full glass of water to minimize esophageal ulceration.
16. For use in pregnancy and in children <8 years old.
17. B Lell and PG Kremsner, Antimicrob Agents Chemother 2002; 46:2315; M Ramharter et al, Clin Infect Dis 2005; 40:1777.
18. At this dosage, adverse effects include nausea, vomiting, diarrhea and dizziness. Disturbed sense of balance, ringing of the ears, toxic psychosis (and other psychiatric effects) and seizures can also occur. Mefloquine can be used for treatment of malaria in pregnant women. The FDA reclassified mefloquine to pregnancy category B based on a review of published data (P Schlagenhauf et al, Clin Infect Dis 2012; 54:e124). It should be avoided for treatment of malaria in persons with active depression or with a history of psychosis or seizures and should be used with caution in persons with any psychiatric illness. Mefloquine should not be used in patients with conduction abnormalities; it can be given to patients taking β-blockers if they do not have an underlying arrhythmia. Mefloquine should not be given together with quinine or quinidine, and caution is required in using quinine or quinidine to treat patients with malaria who have taken mefloquine for prophylaxis. Mefloquine should not be taken on an empty stomach; it should be taken with at least 8 oz of water.
19. *P. falciparum* with resistance to mefloquine is a significant problem in the malarious areas of Thailand and in areas of Myanmar and Cambodia that border on Thailand. It has also been reported on the borders between Myanmar and China, Laos and Myanmar, and in Southern Vietnam. In the US, a 250-mg tablet of mefloquine contains 228 mg mefloquine base. Outside the US, each 275-mg tablet contains 250 mg base.

(continued)

MALARIA, Treatment of (continued)

20. Primaquine phosphate can cause hemolytic anemia, especially in patients whose red cells are deficient in G6PD. This deficiency is most common in African, Asian and Mediterranean peoples. Patients should be screened for G6PD deficiency before treatment. Limited evidence suggests G6PD-deficient patients may be safely treated with a single weekly dose of primaquine 0.75 mg/kg for 8 weeks. Resistance is not known to occur at a dose of 0.5 mg/kg daily for 14 days: suspected resistant strains may be treated with this daily dose for 28 days. Relapse despite adherence to a full primaquine dose may be due to a poor metabolizer phenotype. Primaquine should not be used during pregnancy. It should be taken with food to minimize nausea and abdominal pain.
21. Combination therapy with dihydroartemisinin/piperaquine (*Euartesim*, Sigma-Tau) plus primaquine has demonstrated safety, efficacy and tolerability for treatment of *P. vivax* (I Sutanto et al, Antimicrob Agents Chemother 2013; 57:1128).
22. Medical Letter consultants recommend this combination. Published data on safety or efficacy for cure of *P. vivax* is lacking (JK Baird et al, Antimicrob Agent Chemother 2011; 55:1827).
23. Chloroquine should be taken with food to decrease gastrointestinal adverse effects. If chloroquine phosphate is not available, hydroxychloroquine sulfate is as effective; 400 mg of hydroxychloroquine sulfate is equivalent to 500 mg of chloroquine phosphate.
24. Exchange transfusion is controversial, but has been helpful for some patients with high-density (>10%) parasitemia, altered mental status, pulmonary edema or renal complications (PJ Van Genderen et al, Transfusion 2009; Nov 20 epub).
25. Continuous EKG, blood pressure and glucose monitoring are recommended. Quinine IV is not available in the US. Quinidine may have greater antimalarial activity than quinine. The loading dose should be decreased or omitted in patients who have received quinine or mefloquine. If more than 48 hours of parenteral treatment is required, the quinine or quinidine dose should be reduced by 30-50%. Intrarectal quinine has been tried for the treatment of cerebral malaria in children (J Achan et al, Clin Infect Dis 2007; 45:1446).
26. Oral artesunate is not available in the US; the IV formulation is available through the CDC Malaria branch (M-F 9am-5pm ET, 770-488-7788 or 855-856-4713, or after hours, 770-488-7100) under an IND for patients with severe disease who do not have timely access, cannot tolerate, or fail to respond to IV quinidine (Med Lett Drugs Ther 2008; 50:37). To avoid development of resistance, adults treated with artesunate must also receive oral treatment doses of either atovaquone/proguanil, doxycycline, clindamycin or mefloquine; children should take either atovaquone/proguanil, clindamycin or mefloquine (F Nosten et al, Lancet 2000; 356:297; M van Vugt, Clin Infect Dis 2002; 35:1498; F Smithuis et al, Trans R Soc Trop Med Hyg 2004; 98:182). If artesunate is given IV, oral medication should be started when the patient is able to tolerate it (SEAQUAMAT group, Lancet 2005; 366:717; PE Duffy and CH Sibley, Lancet 2005; 366:1908). Reduced susceptibility to artesunate characterized by slow parasitic clearance has been reported in Cambodia (WO Rogers et al, Malaria J 2009; 8:10; AM Dundorp et al, N Engl J Med 2009; 361:455).

MALARIA, Prevention of[1]

	Drug	Adult dosage	Pediatric dosage
All *Plasmodium* species in chloroquine-resistant areas[2-5]			
Drug of choice:	Atovaquone/ proguanil[6,7]	1 adult tab/d[8]	5-8kg: ½ peds tab/d[7,8] 9-10kg: ¾ peds tab/d[7,8] 11-20kg: 1 peds tab/d[7,8] 21-30kg: 2 peds tabs/d[7,8] 31-40kg: 3 peds tabs/d[7,8] >40kg: 1 adult tab/d[7,8]
OR	Doxycycline[6,9,10]	100 mg PO daily[11]	2 mg/kg/d PO, up to 100 mg/d[11]
OR	Mefloquine[6,12,13]	250 mg PO once/wk[14]	≤ 9kg: 5 mg/kg salt once/wk[14] 9-19kg: ¼ tab once/wk[14] >19-30kg: ½ tab once/wk[14] >31-45kg: ¾ tab once/wk[14] >45kg: 1 tab once/wk[14]
Alternative:[15]	Primaquine[16,17] phosphate	30 mg base PO daily	0.5 mg/kg base PO daily
All *Plasmodium* species in chloroquine-sensitive areas[2-5]			
Drug of choice:[6,18]	Chloroquine phosphate[6,19,20]	500 mg (300 mg base) PO once/wk[21]	5 mg/kg base PO once/wk, up to adult dose of 300 mg base[21]

1. No drug guarantees protection against malaria. Travelers should be advised to seek medical attention if fever develops after they return. Insect repellents, insecticide-impregnated bed nets and proper clothing are important adjuncts for malaria prophylaxis (Treat Guidel Med Lett 2009; 7:83). Malaria in pregnancy is particularly serious for both mother and fetus; prophylaxis is indicated if exposure cannot be avoided.
2. Chloroquine-resistant *P. falciparum* occurs in all malarious areas except Central America (including Panama north and west of the Canal Zone), Mexico, Haiti, the Dominican Republic, Paraguay, northern Argentina, North and South Korea, Georgia, Armenia, most of rural China and some countries in the Middle East (chloroquine resistance has been reported in Yemen, Saudi Arabia and Iran).

(continued)

MALARIA, Prevention of (continued)

3. Chloroquine-resistant *P. vivax* is a significant problem in Papua-New Guinea and Indonesia. There are also reports of resistance from Myanmar, Vietnam, Korea, India, the Solomon Islands, Vanuatu, Indonesia, Guyana, Brazil, Colombia and Peru (JK Baird, Clin Microbiol Rev 2009; 22:508).
4. Chloroquine-resistant *P. malariae* has been reported from Sumatra (JD Maguire et al, Lancet 2002; 360:58).
5. Human infection with the simian species, *P. knowlesi* has been reported in Malaysia where it was initially misdiagnosed as *P. malariae*. Additional cases have been reported from Thailand, Myanmar, Singapore, the Thai-Burma border, and the Philippines (J Cox-Singh et al, Clin Infect Dis 2008; 46:165; MMWR 2009; 58:229).
6. Vivax malaria is a potentially more dangerous infection that previously thought (JK Baird et al, Microbiol Rev 2013; 26:36). Some Medical Letter consultants recommend primaquine as first choice for primary prophylaxis in areas where *P. vivax* is endemic. Atovaquone/proguanil, doxycycline, mefloquine and chloroquine have no activity against latent liver stages of *P. vivax* or *P. ovale*. In one randomized study travelers taking mefloquine (52%) or doxycycline (53%) developed acute *P. vivax* malaria more than a month following travel, while travelers taking daily primaquine had a 6% attack rate (I Schwartz and G Regev-Yochay, Clin Infect Dis 1999; 29:1502). Other Medical Letter consultants prescribe primaquine phosphate 30 mg base/d (0.6 mg base/kg/d for children) in addition to another drug taken during travel for 14d after departure from areas where *P. vivax* or *P. ovale* are endemic (Presumptive Anti-Relapse Therapy [PART]). Since this is not always effective for prevention (E Schwartz et al, N Engl J Med 2003; 349:1510), still others prefer to rely on surveillance to detect cases when they occur, particularly when exposure was limited or doubtful. See also footnote 17.
7. Atovaquone/proguanil is available as a fixed-dose combination tablet: adult tablets (*Malarone*; atovaquone 250 mg/proguanil 100 mg) and pediatric tablets (*Malarone Pediatric*; atovaquone 62.5 mg/proguanil 25 mg). To enhance absorption and reduce nausea and vomiting, it should be taken with food or a milky drink. Safety in pregnancy is unknown and use is generally not recommended. In a few small studies outcomes were normal in women treated with the combination in the 2nd and 3rd trimester (B Paternak et al, Arch Intern Med 2011; 171:259; AK Boggild et al, Am J Trop Med Hyg 2007; 76:208). The drug should not be given to patients with severe renal impairment (creatinine clearance <30mL/min). There have been isolated case reports of resistance in *P. falciparum* in Africa, but Medical Letter consultants do not believe there is a high risk for acquisition of *Malarone*-resistant disease (E Schwartz et al, Clin Infect Dis 2003; 37:450; A Farnert et al, BMJ 2003; 326:628; S Kuhn et al, Am J Trop Med Hyg 2005; 72:407; CT Happi et al, Malaria Journal 2006; 5:82).
8. Beginning 1-2 d before travel and continuing for the duration of stay and for 1wk after leaving malarious zone. In one study of malaria prophylaxis, atovaquone/proguanil was better tolerated than mefloquine in nonimmune travelers (D Overbosch et al, Clin Infect Dis 2001; 33:1015). The protective efficacy of *Malarone* against *P. vivax* is variable ranging from 84% in Indonesian New Guinea (J Ling et al, Clin Infect Dis 2002; 35:825) to 100% in Colombia (J Soto et al, Am J Trop Med Hyg 2006; 75:430). Some Medical Letter consultants prefer alternate drugs if traveling to areas where *P. vivax* predominates.

9. Use of tetracyclines is contraindicated in pregnancy and in children <8 years old. Tetracycline should be taken 1 hour before or 2 hours after meals and/or dairy products.
10. Doxycycline should be taken with adequate water to avoid esophageal irritation. It can be taken with food to minimize gastrointestinal adverse effects.
11. Beginning 1-2 d before travel and continuing for the duration of stay and for 4wks after leaving malarious zone. Doxycycline can cause gastrointestinal disturbances, vaginal moniliasis and photosensitivity reactions.
12. *P. falciparum* with resistance to mefloquine is a significant problem in the malarious areas of Thailand and in areas of Myanmar and Cambodia that border on Thailand. It has also been reported on the borders between Myanmar and China, Laos and Myanmar, and in Southern Vietnam. In the US, a 250-mg tablet of mefloquine contains 228 mg mefloquine base. Outside the US, each 275-mg tablet contains 250 mg base.
13. Mefloquine can be used during pregnancy. The FDA reclassified mefloquine to pregnancy category B based on a review of published data (P Schlagenhauf et al, Clin Infect Dis 2012; 54:e124). It is not recommended for use in travelers with active depression or with a history of psychosis or seizures and should be used with caution in persons with psychiatric illness. Mefloquine should not be used in patients with conduction abnormalities; it can be given to patients taking β-blockers if they do not have an underlying arrhythmia.
14. Beginning 1-2 wks before travel and continuing weekly for the duration of stay and for 4wks after leaving malarious zone. Most adverse events occur within 3 doses. Some Medical Letter consultants favor starting mefloquine 3 weeks prior to travel and monitoring the patient for adverse events, this allows time to change to an alternative regimen if mefloquine is not tolerated. Mefloquine should not be taken on an empty stomach; it should be taken with at least 8 oz of water. For pediatric doses <½ tablet, it is advisable to have a pharmacist crush the tablet, estimate doses by weighing, and package them in gelatin capsules. There is no data for use in children <5 kg, but based on dosages in other weight groups, a dose of 5 mg/kg can be used.
15. The combination of weekly chloroquine (300 mg base) and daily proguanil (200 mg) is recommended by the World Health Organization (www.WHO.int) for use in selected areas; this combination is no longer recommended by the CDC. Proguanil (*Paludrine* – AstraZeneca, United Kingdom) is not available alone in the US but is widely available in Canada and Europe. Prophylaxis is recommended during exposure and for 4 weeks afterwards. Proguanil has been used in pregnancy without evidence of toxicity (PA Phillips-Howard and D Wood, Drug Saf 1996; 14:131).
16. Not FDA-approved for this indication.

(continued)

MALARIA, Prevention of (continued)

17. Primaquine used as primary prophylaxis has proven good safety, tolerability and efficacy when used in non-pregnant, G6PD-normal travelers (DR Hill et al, Am J Trop Med Hyg 2006; 75: 402-15). Beginning the day of travel and for 5 days following travel, this regimen prevents primary attacks of *P. falciparum* and *P. vivax*, and of secondary attacks (relapses) by *P. vivax* in the months following travel. Primaquine can cause hemolytic anemia, especially in patients whose red cells are deficient in G6PD. This deficiency is most common in African, Asian and Mediterranean peoples. Patients should be screened for G6PD deficiency before treatment. Limited evidence suggests G6PD-deficient patients may be safely treated with a single weekly dose of primaquine 0.75 mg/kg for 8 weeks. Resistance is not known to occur at a dose of 0.5 mg/kg daily for 14 days: suspected resistant strains may be treated with this daily dose for 28 days. Relapse despite adherence to a full primaquine dose may be due to a poor metabolizer phenotype. Primaquine should not be used during pregnancy. It should be taken with food to minimize nausea and abdominal pain.
18. Alternatives for patients who are unable to take chloroquine include atovaquone/proguanil, mefloquine, doxycycline or primaquine dosed as for chloroquine-resistant areas.
19. Chloroquine should be taken with food to decrease gastrointestinal adverse effects. If chloroquine phosphate is not available, hydroxychloroquine sulfate is as effective; 400 mg of hydroxychloroquine sulfate is equivalent to 500 mg of chloroquine phosphate.
20. Has been used extensively and safely for prophylaxis in pregnancy.
21. Beginning 1-2 wks before travel and continuing weekly for the duration of stay and for 4 wks after leaving malarious zone.

MALARIA, Self-Presumptive Treatment[1]

		Drug	Adult dosage	Pediatric dosage
Drug of Choice:		Atovaquone/ proguanil[2,3]	4 adult tabs once/d or 2 adult tabs bid x 3d[4]	<5kg: not indicated 5-8kg: 2 peds tabs once/d x 3d 9-10kg: 3 peds tabs once/d x 3d 11-20kg: 1 adult tab once/d x 3d 21-30kg: 2 adult tabs once/d x 3d 31-40kg: 3 adult tabs once/d x 3d >40kg: 4 adult tabs once/d x 3d[4]
	OR	Artemether/ lumefantrine[2,5,6]	6 doses over 3d (4 tabs/dose at 0, 8, 24, 36, 48 and 60 hours)	6 doses over 3d at same intervals as adults; 5-15kg: 1 tab/dose 15-25kg: 2 tabs/dose 25-35kg: 3 tabs/dose >35kg: 4 tabs/dose
	OR	Quinine sulfate	650 mg PO q8h x 3 or 7d[7,8]	30 mg/kg/d PO in 3 doses x 3 or 7d[7]
		plus		
		doxycycline[2,9,10]	100 mg PO bid x 7d	4 mg/kg/d PO in 2 doses x 7d

1. A traveler can be given a course of medication for presumptive self-treatment of febrile illness. The drug given for self-treatment should be different from that used for prophylaxis. This approach should be used only in very rare circumstances when a traveler would not be able to get medical care promptly.
2. Not FDA-approved for this indication.

(continued)

MALARIA, Self-Presumptive Treatment (continued)

3. Atovaquone/proguanil is available as a fixed-dose combination tablet: adult tablets (*Malarone*; atovaquone 250 mg/proguanil 100 mg) and pediatric tablets (*Malarone Pediatric*; atovaquone 62.5 mg/proguanil 25 mg). To enhance absorption and reduce nausea and vomiting, it should be taken with food or a milky drink. Safety in pregnancy is unknown and use is generally not recommended. In a few small studies outcomes were normal in women treated with the combination in the 2nd and 3rd trimester (B Pasternak et al, Arch Intern Med 2011; 171:259; AK Boggild et al, Am J Trop Med Hyg 2007; 76:208). The drug should not be given to patients with severe renal impairment (creatinine clearance <30mL/min). There have been isolated case reports of resistance in *P. falciparum* in Africa, but Medical Letter consultants do not believe there is a high risk for acquisition of *Malarone*-resistant disease (E Schwartz et al, Clin Infect Dis 2003; 37:450; A Farnert et al, BMJ 2003; 326:628; S Kuhn et al, Am J Trop Med Hyg 2005; 72:407; CT Happi et al, Malaria Journal 2006; 5:82).
4. Although approved for once-daily dosing, Medical Letter consultants usually divide the dose in two to decrease nausea and vomiting.
5. Artemether is frequently used globally in combination regimens to treat malaria. It is available in oral, parenteral and rectal formulations, but manufacturing standards are not consistent (HA Karunajeewa et al, JAMA 2007; 297:2381; EA Ashley and NJ White, Curr Opin Infect Dis 2005; 18:531). Based on the few studies available, artemesin derivatives have been relatively safe during pregnancy (I Adam et al, Am Trop Med Parisitol 2009; 103; 205; C Manyando et al, Malaria J 2012; 11:141), but some experts would not prescribe them in the 1st trimester (RL Clark, Reprod Toxicol 2009; 28:285).
6. Artemether/lumefantrine is available as a fixed-dose combination tablet (*Coartem* in the US and in countries with endemic malaria, *Riamet* in Europe and countries without endemic malaria); each tablet contains artemether 20 mg and lumefantrine 120 mg. It is FDA-approved for treatment of uncomplicated malaria and should not be used for severe infection or for prophylaxis. The tablets should be taken with fatty food (tablets may be crushed and mixed with 1-2 tsp water, and taken with milk). Artemether/lumefantrine should not be used in patients with cardiac arrhythmias, bradycardia, severe cardiac disease or QT prolongation. Concomitant use of drugs that prolong the QT interval or are metabolized by CYP2D6 is contraindicated (Med Lett Drugs Ther 2009; 51:75).
7. For treatment of multiple-drug-resistant *P. falciparum* in Southeast Asia, especially Thailand, where mefloquine resistance is frequent, atovaquone/proguanil, quinine plus either doxycycline or clindamycin, or artemether/lumefantrine may be used. For infections acquired elsewhere treatment can be given for 3d.
8. Available in the US in a 324-mg capsule; 2 capsules suffice for adult dosage. In Southeast Asia, relative resistance to quinine has increased and treatment should be continued for 7d. Quinine should be taken with or after meals to decrease gastrointestinal adverse effects. It is generally considered safe in pregnancy.
9. Use of tetracyclines is contraindicated in pregnancy and in children <8 years old. Tetracycline should be taken 1 hour before or 2 hours after meals and/or dairy products.
10. Doxycycline should be taken with adequate water to avoid esophageal irritation. It can be taken with food to minimize gastrointestinal adverse effects.

MICROSPORIDIOSIS

	Drug	Adult dosage	Pediatric dosage
Ocular *(Encephalitozoon hellem, E. cuniculi, Vittaforma [Nosema] corneae)*			
Drug of choice:	Fumagillin[1*]		
	plus		
	albendazole[2,3]	400 mg PO bid	15 mg/kg/d in 2 doses (max 400 mg/dose)
Intestinal *(E. bieneusi, E. [Septata] intestinalis)*			
E. bieneusi			
Drug of choice:	Fumagillin[4*]	20 mg PO tid x 14d	
E. intestinalis			
Drug of choice:	Albendazole[2,3]	400 mg PO bid x 21d	15 mg/kg/d in 2 doses (max 400 mg/dose)
Disseminated (*E. hellem, E. cuniculi, E. intestinalis, Pleistophora sp., Trachipleistophora spp.* and *Anncaliia [Brachiola] vesicularum*)			
Drug of choice:[5]	Albendazole[2,3]	400 mg PO bid	15 mg/kg/d in 2 doses (max 400 mg/dose)

* Availability problems. See table of manufacturers on pages 83-86.

1. CM Chan et al, Ophthalmology 2003; 110:1420. Ocular lesions due to *E. hellem* in HIV-infected patients have responded to fumagillin eyedrops prepared from *Fumidil-B* (bicyclohexyl ammonium fumagillin) used to control a microsporidial disease of honey bees (MJ Garvey et al, Ann Pharmacother 1995; 29:872), available from Leiter's Park Avenue Pharmacy, San Jose, CA (800-292-6773; www.leiterrx.com), a compounding pharmacy that specializes in ophthalmic drugs. For lesions due to *V. corneae*, topical therapy is generally not effective and keratoplasty may be required (RM Davis et al, Ophthalmology 1990; 97:953).
2. Not FDA-approved for this indication.
3. Albendazole must be taken with food; a fatty meal increases oral bioavailability.

(continued)

MICROSPORIDIOSIS (continued)

4. Oral fumagillin (*Flisint* – Sanofi-Aventis, France) has been effective in treating *E. bieneusi* in patients with HIV or solid organ transplants (JM Molina et al, N Engl J Med 2002; 346:1963; F Lanternier et al, Transpl Infect Dis 2009; 11:83), but has been associated with thrombocytopenia and neutropenia. Potent antiretroviral therapy (ART) may lead to microbiologic and clinical response in HIV-infected patients with microsporidial diarrhea. Octreotide *(Sandostatin)* has provided symptomatic relief in some patients with large-volume diarrhea.
5. JM Molina et al, J Infect Dis 1995; 171:245. There is no established treatment for *Pleistophora*. For disseminated disease due to *Trachipleistophora* or *Anncaliia,* itraconazole 400 mg PO once/d plus albendazole may also be tried (CM Coyle et al, N Engl J Med 2004; 351:42).

Mites

See SCABIES

MONILIFORMIS moniliformis infection[1]

	Drug	Adult dosage	Pediatric dosage
Drug of choice:	Pyrante pamoate[2,3]	11 mg/kg base PO once, repeat twice, 2wks apart	11 mg/kg base PO once, repeat twice, 2 wks apart

1. AF Messina et al, Pediatr Infect Dis 2011; 30:728.
2. Not FDA-approved for this indication.
3. Available without a prescription. Pyrantel pamoate suspension can be mixed with milk or fruit juice.

NAEGLERIA species

See AMEBIC MENINGOENCEPHALITIS, PRIMARY

NECATOR americanus

See HOOKWORM infection

OESOPHAGOSTOMUM bifurcum[1]

	Drug	Adult dosage	Pediatric dosage
Drug of choice:	Albendazole	400 mg PO once	15 mg/kg PO once (max 400 mg)
OR	Pyrantel pamoate[2,3]	11 mg/kg base (max 1 g) PO once/d x 3d	11 mg/kg base (max 1 g) PO once/d x 3d

1. JB Ziem et al, Ann Trop Med Parasitol 2004; 98:385.
2. Available without a prescription. Pyrantel pamoate suspension can be mixed with milk or fruit juice.
3. Not FDA-approved for this indication.

ONCHOCERCA volvulus

See FILARIASIS

OPISTHORCHIS viverrini

See FLUKE infection

PARAGONIMUS westermani

See FLUKE infection

PEDICULUS captis, humanus, Phthirus pubis

See LICE

PINWORM

See ENTEROBIUS

PNEUMOCYSTIS jirovecii (formerly *carinii*) pneumonia (PCP)[1]

	Drug	Adult dosage	Pediatric dosage
Moderate to severe disease[2]			
Drug of choice:	Trimethoprim/ sulfamethoxazole	TMP 15-20 mg/kg/d/SMX 75-100 mg/kg/d PO or IV in 3 or 4 doses (change to PO after clinical improvement) x 21d	TMP 15-20 mg/kg/d/SMX 75-100 mg/kg/d PO or IV in 3 or 4 doses (change to PO after clinical improvement) x 21d
Alternative:	Pentamidine	3-4 mg/kg IV daily x 21d	3-4 mg/kg IV daily x 21d
OR	Primaquine[3,4]	30 mg base PO daily x 21d	0.3 mg/kg base PO (max 30 mg) daily x 21d
	plus clindamycin[3,5]	600-900 mg IV tid or qid x 21d, or 300-450 mg PO tid or qid x 21d (change to PO after clinical improvement)	15-25 mg/kg IV tid or qid (max 600 mg/dose) x 21d, or 10 mg/kg PO tid or qid (max 300-450 mg/dose) x 21d (change to PO after clinical improvement)
Mild to moderate disease			
Drug of choice:	Trimethoprim/ sulfamethoxazole	2 DS tablets (160 mg/800 mg each) PO tid x 21d	TMP 15-20 mg/kg/d/SMX 75-100 mg/kg/d PO in 3 or 4 doses x 21d
Alternative:	Dapsone[3]	100 mg PO daily x 21d	2 mg/kg/d (max 100 mg) PO x 21d
	plus trimethoprim[3]	15 mg/kg/d PO in 3 doses	15 mg/kg/d PO in 3 doses
OR	Primaquine[3,4]	30 mg base PO daily x 21d	0.3 mg/kg base PO daily (max 30 mg) x 21d
	plus clindamycin[3,5]	300-450 mg PO tid or qid x 21d	10 mg/kg PO tid or qid (max 300-450 mg/dose) x 21d

(continued)

PNEUMOCYSTIS jirovecii **(formerly *carinii*) pneumonia (PCP) (continued)**				
	OR	Atovaquone[6]	750 mg PO bid x 21d	1-3 mos: 30 mg/kg/d PO in 2 doses x 21d 4-24 mos: 45 mg/kg/d PO in 2 doses x 21d >24 mos: 30 mg/kg/d PO in 2 doses x 21d
Primary and secondary prophylaxis[7]				
Drug of choice:		Trimethoprim/ sulfamethoxazole	1 tab (SS or DS) daily or 1 DS tab PO 3d/wk	TMP 150 mg/SMX 750 mg/m²/d PO in 2 doses 3d/wk
Alternative:		Dapsone[3]	50 mg PO bid or 100 mg PO daily	≥1 mos: 2 mg/kg/d (max 100 mg) PO or 4 mg/kg (max 200 mg) PO once/wk
	OR	Dapsone[3]	50 mg PO daily or 200 mg PO each wk	
		plus pyrimethamine[8]	50 mg PO daily or 75 mg PO each wk	
	OR	Atovaquone[3,6]	1500 mg/d PO in 1 or 2 doses	1-3 mos: 30 mg/kg/d PO 4-24 mos: 45 mg/kg/d PO >24 mos: 30 mg/kg/d PO
	OR	Pentamidine	300 mg aerosol inhaled monthly via *Respirgard II* nebulizer	≥5 yrs: 300 mg inhaled monthly via *Respirgard II* nebulizer

1. Pneumocystis has been reclassified as a fungus (SA Gilroy and NJ Bennett, Semin Respir Crit Care Med 2011; 32:775).
2. In severe disease with room air $PO_2 \leq 70$ mmHg or Aa gradient ≥ 35 mmHg, prednisone or its IV equivalent should also be used. For adults: d 1-5: 40 mg PO bid; d 6-10: 40 mg PO daily; d 11-21: 20 mg PO daily. For children: d 1-5: 2 mg/kg/d PO in 2 doses; d 6-10: 1 mg/kg/d PO in 2 doses; d 11-21: 0.5 mg/kg/d PO daily [JE Kaplan et al, Morbid Mortal Wkly Rep 2009; 58(RR04):1; Morbid Mortal Wkly Rep 2009; 58(RR11):1].
3. Not FDA-approved for this indication.

4. Primaquine phosphate can cause hemolytic anemia, especially in patients deficient in G6PD. This deficiency is most common in African, Asian and Mediterranean peoples. Patients should be screened for G6PD deficiency before treatment. Primaquine should not be used during pregnancy. It should be taken with food to minimize nausea and abdominal pain.
5. Oral clindamycin should be taken with a full glass of water to minimize esophageal ulceration.
6. Atovaquone is available in an oral suspension that should be taken with a meal to increase absorption.
7. Primary/secondary prophylaxis in patients with HIV can be discontinued after CD4 count increases to $>200 \times 10^6$/L for >3mos.
8. Plus leucovorin 25 mg with each dose of pyrimethamine. Pyrimethamine should be taken with food to minimize gastrointestinal adverse effects.

RIVER BLINDNESS

See FILARIASIS

ROUNDWORM

See ASCARIASIS

SARCOCYSTIS spp. (intestinal and muscular)

	Drug	Adult dosage	Pediatric dosage
Drug of choice:	Sarcocystis in humans is acquired by ingesting sporocysts in infected meat. Infection is characterized by nausea, abdominal pain and diarrhea. Most muscle infections are mild or subclinical, although severe and prolonged muscle pain has been reported.[1] Albendazole was reported to be efficacious.[2]		

1. R Fayer, Clin Microbiol Rev 2004; 17:894; MMWR Morb Mortal Wkly Rep 2012; 61:37.
2. MK Arness et al, Am J Trop Med Hyg 1999; 61:548.

SCABIES *(Sarcoptes scabiei)*[1]

	Drug	Adult dosage	Pediatric dosage
Drug of choice:	5% Permethrin	Topically, 2x at least 7 d apart	Topically, 2x at least 7 d apart
Alternative:	Ivermectin[2,3]	200 mcg/kg PO 2x at least 7 d apart[4]	200 mcg/kg PO, 2x at least 7 d apart[4]
	10% Crotamiton	Topically overnight on days 1, 2, 3, 8	Topically overnight on days 1, 2, 3, 8

1. TL Meinking et al, Infestations in LA Schachner and RC Hansen, eds. *Pediatric Dermatology*. 4th ed. St Louis: Mosby; 2011, page 1535; RJ Hay et al, Clin Microbiol Infect 2012; 18:313.
2. Not FDA-approved for this indication.
3. P Gonzalez et al, Curr Pharm Biotechnol 2012; 13:1103. Safety of ivermectin in young children (<15 kg) and pregnant women remains to be established; animal studies have shown adverse effects on the fetus (IM el-Ashmawy et al, Res Vet Sci 2011; 90:116). Taking ivermectin with a meal increases its bioavailability (CA Guzzo et al, J Clin Pharmacol 2002; 42:1122).
4. BJ Currie and JS McCarthy, N Engl J Med 2010; 362:717. A second ivermectin dose taken 2 weeks later increased the cure rate to 95%, which is equivalent to that of 5% permethrin (V Usha et al, J Am Acad Dermatol 2000; 42:236). Ivermectin, either alone or in combination with a topical scabicide, is the drug of choice for crusted scabies in immunocompromised patients (P del Giudice, Curr Opin Infect Dis 2004; 15:123).

SCHISTOSOMIASIS *(Bilharziasis)*[1]

	Drug	Adult dosage	Pediatric dosage
S. haematobium			
Drug of choice:	Praziquantel[2,3]	40 mg/kg/d PO in 1 or 2 doses x 1d	40 mg/kg/d PO in 2 doses x 1d
S. intercalatum[4]			
Drug of choice:	Praziquantel[2,3]	40 mg/kg/d PO in 1 or 2 doses x 1d	40 mg/kg/d PO in 2 doses x 1d
S. japonicum			
Drug of choice:	Praziquantel[2,3]	60 mg/kg/d PO in 2 or 3 doses x 1d	60 mg/kg/d PO in 3 doses x 1d
S. mansoni			
Drug of choice:	Praziquantel[2,3]	40 mg/kg/d PO in 1 or 2 doses x 1d	40 mg/kg/d PO in 2 doses x 1d
Alternative:	Oxamniquine[5]*	15 mg/kg PO once[6]	20 mg/kg/d PO in 2 doses x 1d[6]
S. mekongi			
Drug of choice:	Praziquantel[2,3]	60 mg/kg/d PO in 2 or 3 doses x 1d	60 mg/kg/d PO in 3 doses x 1d

* Availability problems. See table of manufacturers on pages 83-86.

1. Praziquantel is the choice worldwide for treatment and prevention of schistomiasis (R Liu et al, Parasit Vectors 2011; 4:201). Artemisinin treatment early after exposure may decrease the risk of acute disease (AG Ross et al, Lancet Infect Dis 2007; 7:218; R Liu et al, Parasitol Res 2012; 110:2071). It was less effective than praziquantel in an open-label trial of 212 children in Kenya (CO Obonyo et al, Lancet Infect Dis 2010; 10:603).
2. Praziquantel should be taken with liquids during a meal.
3. Retreatment in 2-6 weeks increases cure (MJ Doenhoff et al, Curr Opin Infect Dis 2008; 21:659; DJ Gray et al, BMJ 2011; 342:d2651).
4. Geographically restricted to Central Western Africa and the island of São Tomé. Usually a disease of the lower GI tract; there are also case reports of complications including central nervous system, liver and cardiopulmonary involvement (A Murinello et al, GE - J Port Gastrenterol 2006; 13:97).
5. Oxamniquine, which is not available in the US, is generally not as effective as praziquantel. It has been useful, however, in some areas in which praziquantel is less effective (ML Ferrari et al, Bull World Health Organ 2003; 81:190; A Harder, Parasitol Res 2002; 88:395). Oxamniquine is contraindicated in pregnancy. It should be taken after food.
6. In East Africa, the dose should be increased to 30 mg/kg PO, and in Egypt and South Africa to 30 mg/kg/d PO x 2d. Some experts recommend 40-60 mg/kg PO over 2-3d in all of Africa (KC Shekhar, Drugs 1991; 42:379).

SLEEPING SICKNESS

See TRYPANOSOMIASIS

STRONGYLOIDIASIS *(Strongyloides stercoralis)*

	Drug	Adult dosage	Pediatric dosage
Drug of choice:[1]	Ivermectin[2]	200 mcg/kg/d PO x 2d	200 mcg/kg/d PO x 2d
Alternative:	Albendazole[3,4]	400 mg PO bid x 7d	400 mg PO bid x 7d

1. In immunocompromised patients or disseminated disease (strongyloides hyperinfection syndrome) additional doses or use of other drugs may be necessary. Veterinary subcutaneous and enema formulations of ivermectin have been used in severely ill patients with hyperinfection who were unable to take or reliably absorb oral medications (FM Marty et al, Clin Infect Dis 2005; 41:e5; P Lichtenberger et al, Transpl Infect Dis 2009; 11:137).
2. P Gonzalez et al, Curr Pharm Biotechnol 2012; 13:1103. Safety of ivermectin in young children (<15 kg) and pregnant women remains to be established; animal studies have shown adverse effects on the fetus (IM el-Ashmawy et al, Res Vet Sci 2011; 90:116). Taking ivermectin with a meal increases its bioavailability (CA Guzzo et al, J Clin Pharmacol 2002; 42:1122).
3. Not FDA-approved for this indication.
4. Albendazole must be taken with food; a fatty meal increases oral bioavailability.

TAPEWORM infection

	Drug	Adult dosage	Pediatric dosage
Adult (intestinal stage)			
***Diphyllobothrium latum* (fish), *Taenia saginata* (beef), *Taenia solium* (pork), *Dipylidium caninum* (dog)**			
Drug of choice:	Praziquantel[1,2]	5-10 mg/kg PO once	5-10 mg/kg PO once
Alternative:	Niclosamide[3]*	2 g PO once	50 mg/kg PO once
***Hymenolepis nana* (dwarf tapeworm)**			
Drug of choice:	Praziquantel[1,2]	25 mg/kg PO once	25 mg/kg PO once
Alternative:[4]	Niclosamide[3]*	2 g PO daily x 7d	11-34 kg: 1 g PO on d 1 then 500 mg/d PO x 6 days > 34 kg: 1.5 g PO on d 1 then 1 g/d PO x 6 days
Larval (tissue stage)			
***Echinococcus granulosus* (cystic echinococcosis)**			
Treatment of choice:		See footnote 5	
Drug of choice:	Albendazole[6]	15 mg/kg/d (max 800 mg) PO in 2 doses x 1-6 mos	15 mg/kg/d (max 800 mg) PO in 2 doses x 1-6 mos
***Echinococcus multilocularis* (alveolar echinococcosis)**			
Treatment of choice:		See footnote 7	
Drug of choice:	Albendazole[6]	15 mg/kg/d (max 800 mg) PO in 2 doses x ≥2 yrs	
***Taenia solium* (Cysticercosis)**			
Treatment of choice:		See footnote 8	
Alternative:	Albendazole[6]	15 mg/kg/d (max 800 mg) PO in 2 doses x 8-30d; can be repeated as necessary	15 mg/kg/d (max 800 mg) PO in 2 doses x 8-30d; can be repeated as necessary
OR	Praziquantel[1,2]	50 mg/kg/d PO x 15d	50 mg/kg/d PO x 15d

* Availability problems. See table of manufacturers on pages 83-86.

1. Not FDA-approved for this indication.
2. Praziquantel should be taken with liquids during a meal.
3. Niclosamide must be thoroughly chewed or crushed and swallowed with a small amount of water.
4. Nitazoxanide may be an alternative (JJ Ortiz et al, Trans R Soc Trop Med Hyg 2002; 96:193; JC Chero et al, Trans R Soc Trop Med Hyg 2007; 101:203; E Diaz et al, Am J Trop Med Hyg 2003; 68:384).
5. Treatment of uncomplicated hepatic or abdominal cysts is stage-dependent and ranges from surgical resection to watch and wait (E Brunetti et al, Acta Trop 2010; 114:1). Patients may benefit from surgical resection (for larger cysts) or percutaneous drainage of cysts. Percutaneous aspiration-injection-reaspiration (PAIR) with ultrasound guidance plus albendazole therapy (1 week before and for 30 days after) has been effective for management of hepatic hydatid cyst disease (B Golemanov et al, Am J Trop Med Hyg 2011; 84:48; N Gupta et al, J Gastrointest Surg 2011; 15:1829). Praziquantel may also be useful preoperatively or in case of spillage of cyst contents during surgery.
6. Albendazole must be taken with food; a fatty meal increases oral bioavailability.
7. Surgical excision is the only reliable means of cure (but is rarely possible) and should be followed by prolonged albendazole therapy (P Kern, Curr Opin Infect Dis 2010; 23:505). Reports have suggested that in nonresectable cases, long-term (months to years) use of albendazole (400 mg bid) can stabilize and rarely cure infection (P Moro and PM Schantz, Int J Infect Dis 2009; 13:125; F Chappius, Rev Med Suisse 2012; 8:989).
8. Advances in neuroimaging using CT and MRI have facilitated the ability to make an accurate diagnosis (OH Del Brutto, ScientificWorldJournal 2012; 2012:159821; TE Nash and HH Garcia, Nat Rev Neurol 2011; 7:584). Initial therapy for patients with inflamed parenchymal cysticercosis should focus on symptomatic treatment with anti-seizure medication (S Sinha and BS Sharma, J Clin Neurosci 2009; 16:867). Patients with live parenchymal cysts who have seizures should be treated with albendazole together with steroids and an anti-seizure medication (HH Garcia et al, Curr Opin Infect Dis 2011; 24:423). Patients with subarachnoid cysts or giant cysts in the fissures should be treated for at least 30 days (JV Proaño et al, N Engl J Med 2001; 345:879). Surgical intervention (especially neuroendoscopic removal) or CSF diversion followed by albendazole and steroids is indicated for obstructive hydocephalus. Arachnoiditis, vasculitis or cerebral edema is treated with albendazole or praziquantel plus prednisone (60 mg/d) or dexamethasone (4-6 mg/d). Any cysticidal drug may cause irreparable damage when used to treat ocular or spinal cysts, even when corticosteroids are used. An ophthalmic exam should always precede treatment to rule out intraocular cysts.

TOXOCARIASIS

See VISCERAL LARVA MIGRANS

TOXOPLASMOSIS *(Toxoplasma gondii)*

	Drug	Adult dosage	Pediatric dosage
CNS disease[1]			
Drug of choice:	Pyrimethamine[2]	200 mg PO x 1 then 50-75 mg/d PO x 3-6 wks	2 mg/kg/d PO x 2d, then 1 mg/kg/d (max 25 mg/d) x 3-6 wks
	plus		
	sulfadiazine[3]	1-1.5 g PO qid x 3-6 wks	100-200 mg/kg/d divided q6h PO x 3-6 wks
OR	**plus**		
	clindamycin[4,5,6]	1.8-2.4 g/d IV or PO in 3 or 4 doses	5-7.5 mg/kg/d IV or PO in 3 or 4 doses (max 600 mg/dose)
OR	**plus**		
	atovaquone[4,5,7]	1500 mg PO bid	1500 mg PO bid
Alternative:	Trimethoprim/ sulfamethoxazole[4]	TMP 15-20 mg/kg/d/SMX 75-100 mg/kg/d PO or IV in 3 or 4 doses	TMP 15-20 mg/kg/d/SMX 75-100 mg/kg/d PO or IV in 3 or 4 doses
Primary infection in pregnancy			
Treatment of choice:	See footnote 8		

1. Treatment is followed by chronic suppression with lower dosage regimens of the same drugs. In the US, for primary prophylaxis of HIV patients with CD4 <100 x 10^6 cells/L (outside the US, CD4 <200 x 10^6 cells/L), either trimethoprim/sulfamethoxazole, pyrimethamine with dapsone, or atovaquone with or without pyrimethamine can be used (trimethoprim/sulfamethoxazole is generally preferred due to once-daily dosing). Primary or secondary prophylaxis may be discontinued when the CD4 count increases to >200 x 10^6 cells/L for >3 months (MMWR Morb Mortal Wkly Rep 2009; 58 [RR4]:1). In ocular toxoplasmosis with macular involvement, corticosteroids are recommended in addition to antiparasitic therapy (JG Montoya and O Liesenfeld, Lancet 2004; 363:1965).

2. Plus leucovorin 10-25 mg with each dose of pyrimethamine. Pyrimethamine should be taken with food to minimize gastrointestinal adverse effects.
3 Sulfadiazine should be taken on an empty stomach with adequate water.
4. Not FDA-approved for this indication.
5. Clindamycin has been used in combination with pyrimethamine to treat CNS toxoplasmosis in HIV infected patients who developed sulfonamide sensitivity while on sulfadiazine. Atovaquone has also been used to treat sulfonamide-intolerant patients (K Chirgwin et al, Clin Infect Dis 2002; 34:1243).
6. Oral clindamycin should be taken with a full glass of water to minimize esophageal ulceration.
7. Atovaquone is available in an oral suspension that should be taken with a meal to increase absorption.
8. Women who develop toxoplasmosis during the first trimester of pregnancy should be treated with spiramycin (3-4 g/d). After the first trimester, if there is no documented transmission to the fetus, spiramycin can be continued until term. Spiramycin is not currently available in the US but can be obtained at no cost from Aventis through IND from the FDA (301-796-1600) following confirmation of the diagnosis by a recognized laboratory (i.e. Palo Alto Medical Foundation, Toxoplasmosis Laboratory 650-853-4828). If transmission has occurred *in utero*, therapy with pyrimethamine and sulfadiazine should be started. Pyrimethamine is a potential teratogen and should be used only after the first trimester (JG Montoya and JS Remington, Clin Infect Dis 2008; 47:554). Congenitally infected newborns should be treated with pyrimethamine every 2 or 3 days and a sulfonamide daily for about one year (JS Remington et al, Chapter 31 in JS Remington, *Infectious Disease of the Fetus and Newborn Infant*, 7th ed, Philadelphia:Saunders, 2011, page 918).

TRICHINELLOSIS (*Trichinella spiralis* and other *Trichinella* species)

	Drug	Adult dosage	Pediatric dosage
Drug of choice:[1]	Steroids for severe symptoms, e.g.	prednisone 30-60 mg PO daily x10-15 d	
	plus		
	Albendazole[2,3]	400 mg PO bid x 8-14d	400 mg PO bid x 8-14d
Alternative:	Mebendazole[2]	200-400 mg PO tid x 3d, then 400-500 mg tid x 10d	200-400 mg PO tid x 3d, then 400-500 mg tid x 10d

1. B Gottstein et al, Clin Microbiol Rev 2009; 22:127.
2. Not FDA-approved for this indication.
3. Albendazole must be taken with food; a fatty meal increases oral bioavailability.

TRICHOMONIASIS (*Trichomonas vaginalis*)

	Drug	Adult dosage	Pediatric dosage
Drug of choice:[1]	Tinidazole[2]	2 g PO once	50 mg/kg once (max 2 g)
OR	Metronidazole[3]	2 g PO once	15 mg/kg/d PO in 3 doses x 7d

1. Sexual partners should be treated simultaneously with same dosage. If treatment failure occurs with metronidazole 2 g single dose and reinfection is excluded, treat with metronidazole 500 mg PO bid x7 d. For patients taking 7 d of metronidazole, metronidazole or tinidazole 2 g PO daily x 5 days should be considered. Consultation and susceptibility testing is available from the CDC 404-718-4141 [MMWR Morbid Mortal Wkly Rep 2010; 59(RR-12):1].
2. A nitroimidazole similar to metronidazole, tinidazole appears to be at least as effective as metronidazole and better tolerated. It should be taken with food to minimize GI adverse effects. For children and patients unable to take tablets, a pharmacist can crush the tablets and mix them with cherry syrup (*Humco*, and others). The syrup suspension is good for 7 days at room temperature and must be shaken before use (HB Fung and TL Doan, Clin Ther 2005; 27:1859). Ornidazole, a similar drug, is also used outside the US.
3. Metronidazole has been associated with higher rates of parasitologic and clinical failure compared to tinidazole (LH Bachmann et al, Clin Infect Dis 2011; 53[Suppl 3]:S160).

TRICHOSTRONGYLUS infection

	Drug	Adult dosage	Pediatric dosage
Drug of choice:	Pyrantel pamoate[1,2]	11 mg/kg base PO once (max 1 g)	11 mg/kg base PO once (max 1 g)
Alternative:	Mebendazole[1]	100 mg PO bid x 3d	100 mg PO bid x 3d
OR	Albendazole[1,3]	400 mg PO once	400 mg PO once

1. Not FDA-approved for this indication.
2. Available without a prescription. Pyrantel pamoate suspension can be mixed with milk or fruit juice.
3. Albendazole must be taken with food; a fatty meal increases oral bioavailability.

TRICHURIASIS (*Trichuris trichiura,* whipworm)

	Drug	Adult dosage	Pediatric dosage
Drug of choice:	Albendazole[1,2]	400 mg PO x 3d	400 mg PO x 3d
Alternative:	Mebendazole	100 mg PO bid x 3d	100 mg PO bid x 3d
OR	Ivermectin[1,3]	200 mcg/kg/d PO x 3d	200 mcg/kg/d PO x 3d

1. Not FDA-approved for this indication.
2. Albendazole must be taken with food; a fatty meal increases oral bioavailability.
3. P Gonzalez et al, Curr Pharm Biotechnol 2012; 13:1103. Safety of ivermectin in young children (<15 kg) and pregnant women remains to be established; animal studies have shown adverse effects on the fetus (IM el-Ashmawy et al, Res Vet Sci 2011; 90:116). Taking ivermectin with a meal increases its bioavailability (CA Guzzo et al, J Clin Pharmacol 2002; 42:1122).
4. Ivermectin alone is less effective than albendazole or mebendazole. Addition of ivermectin to albendazole or mebendazole improved cure rates in one study (S Knopp et al, Clin Infect Dis 2010; 51:1420).

TRYPANOSOMIASIS

	Drug	Adult dosage	Pediatric dosage
T. cruzi (American trypanosomiasis, Chagas' disease)[1]			
Drug of choice:	Benznidazole[2]*	5-7 mg/kg/d PO in 2 doses x 60d	≤12 yrs: 10 mg/kg/d PO in 2 doses x 60d >12 yrs: 5-7 mg/kg/d PO in 2 doses x 60d
OR	Nifurtimox*	8-10 mg/kg/d PO in 3-4 doses x 90d	1-10 yrs: 15-20 mg/kg/d PO in 4 doses x 90d 11-16 yrs: 12.5-15 mg/kg/d PO in 4 doses x 90d
T. brucei gambiense (West African trypanosomiasis, sleeping sickness)[3]			
Hemolymphatic stage			
Drug of choice:[4]	Pentamidine[5]	4 mg/kg/d IM or IV x 7d	4 mg/kg/d IM or IV x 7d
Alternative:	Suramin*	100 mg (test dose) IV, then 1 g IV on days 1,3,5,14 and 21	2 mg/kg (test dose) IV, then 20 mg/kg IV on d 1,3,5,14 and 21
Late disease with CNS involvement			
Drug of choice:[6]	Eflornithine[7]*	400 mg/kg/d IV in 4 doses x 14d	400 mg/kg/d IV in 4 doses x 14d
OR	Eflornithine[7]*	400 mg/kg IV in 2 doses x 7d	
	plus		
	nifurtimox	15 mg/kg/d PO in 3 doses x 10d	
Alternative:	Melarsoprol[8]	2.2 mg/kg/d IV x 10d	2.2 mg/kg/d IV x 10d
T. b. rhodesiense (East African trypanosomiasis, sleeping sickness)[3]			
Hemolymphatic stage			
Drug of choice:	Suramin*	100 mg (test dose) IV, then 1 g IV on days 1,3,5,14 and 21	2 mg/kg (test dose) IV, then 20 mg/kg IV on d 1,3,5,14 and 21
Late disease with CNS involvement			
Drug of choice:	Melarsoprol[8]	2.2 mg/kg/d IV x 10d	2.2 mg/kg/d IV x 10d

* Availability problems. See table of manufacturers on pages 83–86.

1. Treatment of chronic or indeterminate Chagas' disease with benznidazole has been associated with negative seroconversion in children and reduced progression of cardiac disease in adults (R Viotti et al, Ann Intern Med 2006; 144:724; AL de Andrade, Lancet 1996; 348:1407; C Bern et al, Clin Microbiol Rev 2011; 24:655; G LeLoup et al, Curr Opin Infect Dis 2011; 24:428). Congenital transmission of Chagas' disease occurs in 1-10% of children born to infected mothers. The safety of antitrypanasomal drugs in pregnancy is unknown. The treatment of mothers after delivery and cessation of breast feeding is recommended (MMWR Morb Mortal Wkly Rep 2012; 61:477; Y Carlier et al, PLoS Negl Trop Dis 2011; 5:e1250).
2. Benznidazole should be taken with meals to minimize gastrointestinal adverse effects. It is contraindicated during pregnancy.
3. JA Blum et al, Eur J Clin Microbiol Infect Dis 2012; D Malvy and F Chappuis, Clin Microbiol Infect 2011; 17:986.
4. Pentamidine and suramin have equal efficacy, but pentamidine is better tolerated.
5. Not FDA-approved for this indication.
6. In one study, eflornithine for 7 days combined with nifurtimox x 10 days was more effective and less toxic than eflornithine x 14 days (G Priotto et al, Lancet 2009; 374:56).
7. Eflornithine is highly effective in *T.b. gambiense*, but not in *T.b. rhodesiense* infections. In two studies of treatment of CNS disease due to *T.b. gambiense*, there were fewer serious complications with eflornithine than with melarsoprol (PG Kennedy, Ann Neurol 2008; 64:116; F Chappuis et al, Clin Infect Dis 2005; 41:748). Eflornithine is available in limited supply only from the WHO.
8. I Kuepfer et al, PLoS Negl Trop Dis 2012; 6:e1695. Corticosteroids have been used to prevent arsenical encephalopathy (J Pepin et al, Trans R Soc Trop Med Hyg 1995; 89:92).

VISCERAL LARVA MIGRANS[1] *(Toxocariasis)*

	Drug	Adult dosage	Pediatric dosage
Drug of choice:	Albendazole[2,3]	400 mg PO bid x 5d	400 mg PO bid x 5d
OR	Mebendazole[2]	100-200 mg PO bid x 5d	100-200 mg PO bid x 5d

1. Optimum duration of therapy is not known; some Medical Letter consultants would treat x 20 d. For severe symptoms or eye involvement, treatment is extended 2-4 weeks and corticosteroids can be used in addition (G Rubinsky-Elefant et al, Ann Trop Parasitol 2010; 104:3; MC Turrientes et al, Emerg Infect Dis 2011; 17:1263).
2. Not FDA-approved for this indication.
3. Albendazole must be taken with food; a fatty meal increases oral bioavailability.

WHIPWORM

See TRICHURIASIS

WUCHERERIA bancrofti

See FILARIASIS

PRINCIPAL ADVERSE EFFECTS OF ANTIPARASITIC DRUGS

Adverse effects of antiparasitic drugs vary with dosage, duration of administration, concomitant therapy, renal and hepatic function, immune competence, and the age of the patient. The principal adverse effects of antiparasitic agents are listed in the following table. The designation of adverse effects as "frequent," "occasional" or "rare" is based on published reports and on the experience of Medical Letter consultants.

ALBENDAZOLE *(Albenza)*

Frequent: abdominal pain; increased serum transaminases
Occasional: reversible alopecia; leukopenia
Rare: rash; hepatic toxicity; renal toxicity

AMPHOTERICIN B DEOXYCHOLATE (*Fungizone*, and generics)

Frequent: renal damage; hypokalemia; thrombophlebitis at site of peripheral vein infusion; anorexia; headache; nausea; weight loss; bone marrow suppression with reversible decline in hematocrit; chills, fever, vomiting during infusion, possibly with delirium, hypotension or hypertension, wheezing, and hypoxemia, especially in cardiac or pulmonary diease
Occasional: hypomagnesemia; normocytic, normochromic anemia
Rare: hemorrhagic gastroenteritis; blood dyscrasias; rash; blurred vision; peripheral neuropathy; convulsions; anaphylaxis; arrhythmias; acute liver failure; reversible nephrogenic diabetes insipidus; hearing loss; acute pulmonary edema; spinal cord damage with intrathecal use

AMPHOTERICIN B LIPID FORMULATIONS *(AmBisone, Abelcet, Amphotec)*

Similar to amphotericin B but generally better tolerated. Nephrotoxicity is less common and less severe with the lipid-based formulations. Acute infusion reactions are worse with *Amphotec,* less with *Abelcet* and least with *AmBisome.* Liver toxicity has been reported.

ARTEMETHER *(Artenam)*
Occasional: neurological toxicity; possible increase in length of coma; increased convulsions; prolongation of QTc interval

ARTEMETHER/LUMEFANTRINE *(Coatem, Riamet)*
Frequent: abdominal pain; anorexia; headache; dizziness; diarrhea; vomiting; nausea; palpitations; arthralgia; myalgia; asthenia; fatigue; pruritus; rash; sleep disorder; cough
Occasional: somnolence; involuntary muscle contractions; paresthesia; hypoesthesia; abnormal gait; ataxia
Rare: Hypersensitivity

ARTESUNATE
Occasional: ataxia; slurred speech; neurological toxicity; possible increase in length of coma; increased convulsions; prolongation of QTc interval

ATOVAQUONE (*Mepron, Malarone* [with proguanil])
Frequent: rash; nausea
Occasional: diarrhea; increased aminotransferases; cholestasis

AZITHROMYCIN (*Zithromax*, and generics)
Occasional: nausea; diarrhea; abdominal pain; headache; dizziness; vaginitis
Rare: angioedema; cholestatic jaundice; photosensitivity; reversible dose-related hearing loss; QT prolongation

BENZNIDAZOLE *(Rochagan)*
Frequent: allergic rash; dose-dependent polyneuropathy; GI disturbance; psychic disturbances

BENZYL ALCOHOL *(Ulesfia Lotion)*
Frequent: eye irritation; contact dermatitis

BITHIONOL *(Bitin)*
Frequent: photosensitivity reactions; vomiting; diarrhea; abdominal pain; urticaria
Rare: leukopenia; toxic hepatitis

CHLOROQUINE HCL and **CHLOROQUINE PHOSPHATE** (*Aralen,* and generics)
Occasional: pruritus; vomiting; headache; confusion; depigmentation of hair; skin eruptions; corneal opacity; weight loss; partial alopecia; extraocular muscle palsies; exacerbation of psoriasis, eczema, and other exfoliative dermatoses; myalgias; photophobia
Rare: irreversible retinal injury (especially when total dosage exceeds 100 grams); discoloration of nails and mucus membranes; nerve-type deafness; peripheral neuropathy and myopathy; heart block; blood dyscrasias; hematemesis

CLARITHROMYCIN (*Biaxin*, and generics)
Occasional: nausea; diarrhea; abdominal pain; abnormal taste; headache; dizziness
Rare: reversible dose-related hearing loss; pseudomembranous colitis; pancreatitis; torsades de pointes

CLINDAMYCIN (*Cleocin*, and generics)
Frequent: diarrhea; allergic reactions
Occasional: pseudomembranous colitis, sometimes severe, can occur even with topical use
Rare: blood dyscrasias; esophageal ulceration; hepatotoxicity; arrhythmia due to QTc prolongation

CROTAMITON *(Eurax)*
Occasional: rash

DAPSONE

Frequent: rash; transient headache; GI irritation; anorexia; infectious mononucleosis-like syndrome

Occasional: cyanosis due to methemoglobinemia and sulfhemoglobinemia; other blood dyscrasias, including hemolytic anemia; nephrotic syndrome; liver damage; peripheral neuropathy; hypersensitivity reactions; increased risk of lepra reactions; insomnia; irritability; uncoordinated speech; agitation; acute psychosis

Rare: renal papillary necrosis; severe hypoalbuminemia; epidermal necrolysis; optic atrophy; agranulocytosis; neonatal hyperbilirubinemia after use in pregnancy

DIETHYLCARBAMAZINE CITRATE *(Hetrazan)*

Frequent: allergic or febrile reactions, which may be severe, in patients with microfilaria in the blood or the skin; GI disturbance

Rare: encephalopathy

DILOXANIDE FUROATE *(Furamide)*

Frequent: flatulence

Occasional: nausea; vomiting; diarrhea

Rare: diplopia; dizziness; urticaria; pruritus

EFLORNITHINE (Difluoromethylornithine, DFMO, *Ornidyl*)

Frequent: anemia; leukopenia

Occasional: diarrhea; thrombocytopenia; seizures

Rare: hearing loss

FLUCONAZOLE (*Diflucan*, and generics)

Occasional: nausea; vomiting; diarrhea; abdominal pain; headache; rash; increased aminotransferases

Rare: severe hepatic toxicity; exfoliative dermatitis; anaphylaxis; Stevens-Johnson syndrome; toxic epidermal necrolysis; hair loss

FLUCYTOSINE *(Ancobon)*

Frequent: blood dyscrasias, including pancytopenia and fatal agranulocytosis; GI disturbance, including severe diarrhea and ulcerative colitis; rash; hepatic dysfunction

Occasional: confusion; hallucinations

Rare: anaphylaxis

FURAZOLIDONE *(Furoxone)*

Frequent: nausea; vomiting

Occasional: allergic reactions, including pulmonary infiltration; hypotension; urticaria; fever; vesicular rash; hypoglycemia; headache

Rare: hemolytic anemia in G6PD deficiency and neonates; disulfiram-like reaction with alcohol; MAO-inhibitor interactions; polyneuritis

IODOQUINOL (*Yodoxin*, and generics)

Occasional: rash; acne; slight enlargement of the thyroid gland; nausea; diarrhea; cramps; anal pruritus

Rare: optic neuritis, atrophy and loss of vision; peripheral neuropathy after prolonged use in high dosage (for months); iodine sensitivity

ITRACONAZOLE (*Sporanox*, and generics)

Occasional: nausea; epigastric pain; headache; dizziness; edema; hypokalemia; rash; hepatic toxicity

Rare: congestive heart failure

IVERMECTIN – oral *(Stromectol)*

Occasional: Mazzotti-type reaction seen in onchocerciasis, including fever; pruritus; tender lymph nodes; headache; and joint and bone pain

Rare: hypotension

IVERMECTIN – lotion *(Sklice)*

Occasional: conjunctivitis; ocular hyperemia; eye irritation; dandruff; burning sensation of the skin

KETOCONAZOLE (*Nizoral*, and generics)
Frequent: nausea; vomiting
Occasional: decreased testosterone synthesis; gynecomastia; oligospermia and impotence in men; abdominal pain; rash; hepatitis; pruritus; dizziness; constipation; diarrhea; fever and chills; photophobia; headache
Rare: fatal hepatic necrosis; liver injury with jaundice; transient elevated transaminase; severe epigastric burning and pain; may interfere with adrenal function; anaphylaxis

MALATHION *(Ovide)*
Occasional: local irritation

MEBENDAZOLE *(Vermox)*
Occasional: diarrhea; abdominal pain
Rare: leukopenia; agranulocytosis; hypospermia

MEFLOQUINE *(Lariam)*
Frequent: vertigo; lightheadedness; nausea; other GI disturbances; nightmares; visual disturbances; headache; insomnia
Occasional: confusion
Rare: psychosis; hypotension; convulsions; coma; paresthesias

MEGLUMINE ANTIMONIATE *(Glucantime)*
Similar to sodium stibogluconate

MELARSOPROL *(Mel B)*
Frequent: myocardial damage; albuminuria; hypertension; colic; Herxheimer-type reaction; encephalopathy; vomiting; peripheral neuropathy
Rare: shock

METRONIDAZOLE (*Flagyl*, and generics)
Frequent: nausea; headache; anorexia; metallic taste
Occasional: vomiting; diarrhea; insomnia; weakness; dry mouth; stomatitis; vertigo; tinnitus; paresthesias; rash; dark urine; urethral burning; disulfiram-like reaction with alcohol; candidiasis
Rare: pseudomembranous colitis; leukopenia; pancreatitis; seizures; peripheral neuropathy; encephalopathy; cerebellar syndrome with ataxia, dysarthria and MRI abnormalities

MICONAZOLE *(Monistat)*
Occasional: phlebitis; thrombocytosis; chills; intense, persistent pruritus; rash; vomiting; hyperlipidemia; dizziness; blurred vision; local burning and irritation with topical use
Rare: anemia; thrombocytopenia; hyponatremia; renal insufficiency; anaphylaxis; cardiac and respiratory arrest with initial dose

MILTEFOSINE *(Impavido)*
Frequent: nausea; vomiting; diarrhea; motion sickness; increased creatinine

NICLOSAMIDE *(Niclocide)*
Occasional: nausea; abdominal pain

NIFURTIMOX *(Lampit)*
Frequent: anorexia; nausea; vomiting; gastric pain; insomnia; headache; vertigo; excitability; myalgia; arthralgia; peripheral polyneuritis
Rare: convulsions; fever; pulmonary infiltrates; pleural effusion

NITAZOXANIDE *(Alinia)*
Occasional: GI disturbance; headache
Rare: yellow discoloration of sclera; allergic reactions; increased creatinine; dizziness; flatulence; malaise; salivary gland enlargement; discolored urine; anemia; leukoytosis

ORNIDAZOLE *(Tiberal)*
Occasional: dizziness; headache; GI disturbance
Rare: reversible peripheral neuropathy

OXAMNIQUINE *(Vansil)*
Occasional: headache; fever; dizziness; somnolence and insomnia; nausea; diarrhea; rash; increased aminotransferases; ECG changes; EEG changes; orange-red discoloration of urine
Rare: seizures; neuropsychiatric disturbances

PAROMOMYCIN (aminosidine; *Humatin*)
Frequent: GI disturbance with oral use
Rare: eighth-nerve damage (mainly auditory) and renal damage when aminosidine is given IV; vertigo; pancreatitis

PENTAMIDINE ISETHIONATE (*Pentam 300, NebuPent,* and generics)
Frequent: hypotension; hypoglycemia often followed by diabetes mellitus; vomiting; blood dyscrasias; renal damage; pain at injection site; GI disturbance
Occasional: may aggravate diabetes; shock; hypocalcemia; liver damage; cardiotoxicity; delirium; rash
Rare: Herxheimer-type reaction; anaphylaxis; acute pancreatitis; hyperkalemia

PERMETHRIN (*Nix,* and generics)
Occasional: burning; stinging; numbness; increased pruritus; pain; edema; erythema; rash

PRAZIQUANTEL *(Biltricide)*
Frequent: abdominal pain; diarrhea; malaise; headache; dizziness
Occasional: sedation; fever; sweating; nausea; eosinophilia
Rare: pruritus; rash; edema; hiccups

PRIMAQUINE PHOSPHATE
Frequent: hemolytic anemia in G6PD deficiency
Occasional: neutropenia; GI disturbance; methemoglobinemia
Rare: CNS symptoms; hypertension; arrhythmias

PROGUANIL *(Paludrine; Malarone* [with atovaquone])
Occasional: oral ulceration; hair loss; scaling of palms and soles; urticaria
Rare: hematuria (with large doses); vomiting; abdominal pain; diarrhea (with large doses); thrombocytopenia

PYRANTEL PAMOATE (*Antiminth*, and generics)
Occasional: GI disturbance; headache; dizziness; rash; fever

PYRETHRINS with PIPERONYL BUTOXIDE (*A-200*, and generics)
Occasional: allergic reactions

PYRIMETHAMINE *(Daraprim)*
Occasional: blood dyscrasias; folic acid deficiency
Rare: rash; vomiting; convulsions; shock; possibly pulmonary eosinophilia; fatal cutaneous reactions with pyrimethamine/sulfadoxine *(Fansidar)*

QUINACRINE
Frequent: disulfiram-like reaction with alcohol; nausea and vomiting; colors skin and urine yellow
Occasional: headache; dizziness
Rare: rash; fever; psychosis; extensive exfoliative dermatitis in patients with psoriasis

QUININE DIHYDROCHLORIDE and QUININE SULFATE

Frequent: cinchonism (tinnitus, headache, nausea, abdominal pain, visual disturbance)
Occasional: deafness; hemolytic anemia; other blood dyscrasias; photosensitivity reactions; hypoglycemia; arrhythmias; hypotension; fever
Rare: blindness; sudden death if injected too rapidly; hypersensitivity reaction with TTP-HUS

SODIUM STIBOGLUCONATE *(Pentostam)*

Frequent: myalgia and arthralgia (typically, large joint, may or may not be symmetric); malaise, fatigue and weakness; headache; anorexia; nausea; increased aminotransferases; increased amylase and lipase; T-wave flattening or inversion
Occasional: abdominal pain; liver damage; bradycardia; leukopenia; thrombocytopenia; rash; vomiting
Rare: diarrhea; pruritus; myocardial damage; hemolytic anemia; renal damage; shock; sudden death

SPIRAMYCIN *(Rovamycine)*

Occasional: GI disturbance
Rare: allergic reactions

SULFONAMIDES

Frequent: allergic reactions (rash, photosensitivity, drug fever)
Occasional: kernicterus in newborn; renal damage; liver damage; Stevens-Johnson syndrome (particularly with long-acting sulfonamides); hemolytic anemia; other blood dyscrasias; vasculitis
Rare: transient acute myopia; pseudomembranous colitis; reversible infertility in men with sulfasalazine; CNS toxicity with trimethoprim/sulfamethoxazole in patients with AIDS

SURAMIN SODIUM

Frequent: vomiting; pruritus; urticaria; paresthesias; hyperesthesia of hands and feet; peripheral neuropathy; photophobia
Occasional: kidney damage; blood dyscrasias; shock; optic atrophy

TETRACYCLINES
(doxycycline – *Vibramycin*, and generics; tetracycline hydrochloride – *Sumycin*, and generics)

Frequent: GI disturbance; bone lesions and staining and deformity of teeth in children up to 8 years old, and in the newborn when given to pregnant women after the fourth month of pregnancy

Occasional: malabsorption; enterocolitis; photosensitivity reactions; increased azotemia with renal insufficiency (except doxycycline, but exacerbation of renal failure with doxycycline has been reported); hepatic injury; parenteral doses may cause serious liver damage, especially in pregnant women and patients with renal disease receiving 1 gram or more daily; esophageal ulcerations; cutaneous and mucosal hyperpigmentation

Rare: allergic reactions, including serum sickness and anaphylaxis; pseudomembranous colitis; blood dyscrasias; drug-induced lupus; autoimmune hepatitis; increased intracranial pressure; fixed-drug eruptions; transient acute myopia; blurred vision; diplopia; papilledema; photoonycholysis and onycholysis; aggravation of myasthenic symptoms with IV injection, reversed with calcium; possibly transient neuropathy; hemolytic anemia

TINIDAZOLE (*Tindamax*, and generics)

Occasional: metallic taste; GI symptoms; rash

Rare: weakness

TRIMETHOPRIM (*Proloprim*, and generics)

Frequent: nausea and vomiting with high doses

Occasional: megaloblastic anemia; thrombocytopenia; neutropenia; rash; fixed drug eruption

Rare: pancytopenia; hyperkalemia

TRIMETHOPRIM/SULFAMETHOXAZOLE (*Bactrim, Septra*, and generics)

Frequent: rash; fever; nausea and vomiting

Occasional: hemolysis in G6PD deficiency; acute megaloblastic anemia; granulocytopenia; thrombocytopenia; pseudomembranous colitis; kernicterus in newborn; hyperkalemia

Rare: agranulocytosis; aplastic anemia; hepatotoxicity; Stevens-Johnson syndrome; aseptic meningitis; fever; confusion; depression; hallucinations; deterioration in renal disease; intrahepatic cholestasis; methemoglobinemia; pancreatitis; ataxia; CNS toxicity in patients with AIDS; renal tubular acidosis; hyperkalemia

SAFETY OF ANTIPARASITIC DRUGS IN PREGNANCY

Drug	Toxicity in Pregnancy	Recommendations	FDA
Albendazole *(Albenza)*	Teratogenic and embryotoxic in animals	Caution*; contraindicated for long-term use	C
Amphotericin B (*Fungizone*, and generics)	None known	Caution*	B
Amphotericin B liposomal *(AmBisome)*	None known	Caution*	B
Artemether/lumefantrine *(Coartem, Riamet)*[1]	Embryo-fetal loss in rats and rabbits	Contraindicated during 1st trimester; caution 2nd and 3rd trimesters*	C
Artesunate[1]	Embryocidal and teratogenic in rats	Contraindicated during 1st trimester; caution 2nd and 3rd trimesters*	N/A
Atovaquone *(Mepron)*	Maternal and fetal toxicity in animals	Caution*	C
Atovaquone/proguanil *(Malarone)*[2]	Maternal and fetal toxicity in animals	Caution*	C
Azithromycin (*Zithromax*, and generics)	None known	Probably safe	B
Benznidazole *(Rochagan)*	Unknown	Contraindicated	N/A
Benzyl alcohol lotion *(Ulesfia Lotion)*	Unknown	Probably safe	B
Chloroquine (*Aralen*, and generics)	None known with doses recommended for malaria prophylaxis	Probably safe in low doses	C
Clarithromycin (*Biaxin*, and generics)	Teratogenic in animals	Contraindicated	C
Clindamycin (*Cleocin*, and generics)	None known	Caution*	B
Crotamiton *(Eurax)*	Unknown	Caution*	C
Dapsone	None known; carcinogenic in rats and mice; hemolytic reactions in neonates	Caution,* especially at term	C

Diethylcarbamazine (DEC; *Hetrazan*)	Not known; abortifacient in one study in rabbits	Contraindicated	N/A
Diloxanide *(Furamide)*	Safety not established	Caution*	N/A
Doxycycline (*Vibramycin*, and generics)	Tooth discoloration and dysplasia inhibition of bone growth in fetus; hepatic toxicity and azotemia with IV use in pregnant patients with decreased renal function or with overdosage	Contraindicated	D
Eflornithine *(Ornidyl)*	Embryocidal in animals	Contraindicated	C
Fluconazole (*Diflucan*, and generics)	Teratogenic	Contraindicated for high dose; caution* for single dose	C
Flucytosine *(Ancoban)*	Teratogenic in rats	Contraindicated	C
Furazolidone *(Furoxone)*	None known; carcinogenic in rodents; hemolysis with G6PD deficiency in newborn	Caution*; contraindicated at term	N/A
Hydroxychloroquine *(Plaquenil)*	None known with doses recommended for malaria prophylaxis	Probably safe in low doses	C
Itraconazole (*Sporanox*, and generics)	Teratogenic and embryotoxic in rats	Caution*	C
Iodoquinol (*Yodoxin*, and generics)	Unknown	Caution*	C
Ivermectin *(Sklice, Stromectol)*[3]	Teratogenic in animals	Contraindicated	C
Ketoconazole (*Nizoral*, and generics)	Teratogenic and embryotoxic in rats	Contraindicated; topical probably safe	C
Lindane	Absorbed from the skin; potential CNS toxicity in fetus	Contraindicated	C
Malathion, topical *(Ovide)*	None known	Probably safe	B

Drug	Toxicity in Pregnancy	Recommendations	FDA
Mebendazole *(Vermox)*	Teratogenic and embryotoxic in rats	Caution*	C
Mefloquine *(Lariam)*[4]	Teratogenic in animals	Caution*	B
Meglumine *(Glucantine)*	Not known	Caution*	N/A
Metronidazole (*Flagyl*, and generics)	None known – carcinogenic in rats and mice	Caution*	B
Miconazole *(Monistat)*	None known	Caution*	C
Miltefosine *(Impavido)*	Teratogenic in rats and induces abortions inanimals	Contraindicated; effective contraception must be used for 2 months after the last dose	N/A
Niclosamide *(Niclocide)*	Not absorbed; no known toxicity in fetus	Probably safe	B
Nifurtimox *(Lampit)*	Retarded growth in rats and mice	Caution*; contraindicated during 1st trimester	N/A
Nitazoxanide *(Alinia)*	None known	Probably safe	B
Oxamniquine *(Vansil)*	Embryocidal in animals	Contraindicated	N/A
Paromomycin	Poorly absorbed; toxicity in fetus unknown	Oral capsules probably safe	C
Pentamidine (*Pentam 300, NebuPent,* and others)	Safety not established	Caution*	C
Permethrin (*Nix,* and generics)	Poorly absorbed; no known toxicity in fetus	Probably safe	B
Praziquantel *(Biltricide)*	None known	Caution	B
Primaquine	Hemolysis in G6PD deficiency	Contraindicated	C
Pyrantel pamoate (*Antiminth,* and generics)	Absorbed in small amounts; no known toxicity in fetus	Probably safe	C

Pyrethrins and piperonyl butoxide (*A-200*, and generics)	Poorly absorbed; no known toxicity in fetus	Probably safe	C
Pyrimethamine *(Daraprim)*[5]	Teratogenic in animals	Caution*; contraindicated during 1st trimester	C
Quinacrine *(Atabrine)*	Safety not established	Caution*	N/A
Quinidine	Large doses can cause abortion	Probably safe	C
Quinine *(Qualaquin)*	Large doses can cause abortion; auditory nerve hypoplasia, deafness in fetus; visual changes, limb anomalies, visceral defects also reported	Caution*	C
Sodium stibogluconate *(Pentostam)*	Not known	Caution*	N/A
Spiramycin *(Rovamycine)*[5]	None known	Probably safe	N/A
Sulfonamides	Teratogenic in some animal studies; hemolysis in newborn with G6PD deficiency; increased risk of kernicterus in newborn	Caution*; contraindicated at term	C
Suramin sodium *(Germanin)*	Teratogenic in mice	Caution*	N/A
Tetracycline (*Sumycin*, and generics)	Tooth discoloration and dysplasia, inhibition of bone growth in fetus; hepatic toxicity and azotemia with IV use in pregnant patients with decreased renal function or with overdosage	Contraindicated	D
Tinidazole (*Tindamax*, and generics)	Increased fetal mortality in rats	Caution*	C
Trimethoprim	Folate antagonism; teratogenic in rats	Caution*	C

Drug	Toxicity in Pregnancy	Recommendations	FDA
Trimethoprim/sulfamethoxazole (*Bactrim*, and generics)	Same as sulfonamides and trimethoprim	Caution*; contraindicated at term	C

N/A= FDA pregnancy category not available

*Use only for strong clinical indication in absence of suitable alternative.

1. Based on the few studies available, artemesinins have been relatively safe during pregnancy (I Adam et al, Am Trop Med Parisitol 2009; 103:205), but some experts would not prescribe them in the 1st trimester (RL Clark, Reprod Toxicol 2009; 28:285; C Manyando et al, Malaria J 2012; 11:141).
2. Safety in pregnancy is unknown; in a few small studies; outcomes were normal in women treated with the combination in the 2nd and 3rd trimester (AK Boggild et al, Am J Trop Med Hyg 2007; 76:208).
3. Ivermectin has been inadvertently given to pregnant women during mass treatment programs; the rates of congenital abnormalities were similar in treated and untreated women. Because of the high risk of blindness from onchocerciasis, the use of ivermectin after the first trimester is considered acceptable according to the WHO.
4. Mefloquine can be used for prophylaxis or treatment of malaria in pregnant women based on a review of published data (P Schlagenhauf et al, Clin Infect Dis 2012; 54:e124).
5. Women who develop toxoplasmosis during the first trimester of pregnancy should be treated with spiramycin (3-4 g/d). After the first trimester, if there is no documented transmission to the fetus, spiramycin can be continued until term. If transmission has occurred *in utero*, therapy with pyrimethamine and sulfadiazine should be started. Pyrimethamine is a potential teratogen and should be used only after the first trimester (JG Montoya and JS Remington, Clin Infect Dis 2008; 47:554).

MANUFACTURERS OF DRUGS USED TO TREAT PARASITIC INFECTIONS

	Generic Name	Brand Name	Manufacturer
	albendazole	*Albenza*	Amedra
	amphotericin B	Fungizone, generics	X-Gen
	amphotericin B, liposomal	*AmBisome*	Gilead
§	artemether	*Artenam*	Arenco, Belgium
	artemether/lumefantrine	*Coartem, Riamet*	Novartis
†	artesunate		Guilin, Shanghai
	atovaquone	*Mepron*	GlaxoSmithKline
	atovaquone/proguanil	*Malarone*	GlaxoSmithKline
	azithromycin	*Zithromax*, generics	Pfizer
†	benznidazole	*Rochagan*	
§	bithionol	*Bitin*	
	chloroquine	*Aralen*, generics	Sanofi
	clarithromycin	*Biaxin*, generics	Abbvie
	clindamycin	*Cleocin*, generics	Pfizer
	crotamiton	*Eurax*	Ranbaxy
	dapsone	generics	Jacobus
†	diethylcarbamazine citrate (DEC)	*Hetrazan*	
	dihydroartemisin/piperaquine	*Euratesim*	Sigma-Tau, Italy
§	diloxanide furoate	*Furamide, Entamide*	
	doxycycline	*Vibramycin*, generics	Pfizer
†	eflornithine (Difluoromethylornithine, DFMO)	*Ornidyl*	Sanofi
	fluconazole	*Diflucan*, generics	Pfizer

	Generic Name	Brand Name	Manufacturer
	flucytosine	*Ancobon*	Valeant
§	fumagillin	*Flisint*	Sanofi, France
§	furazolidone	*Furoxone*	
	iodoquinol	*Yodoxin*, generics	Glenwood
	itraconazole	*Sporanox*, generics	Janssen
	ivermectin	*Stromectol*	Merck
		Sklice	Sanofi
	ketoconazole	*Nizoral*, generics	Janssen
	lumefantrine/artemether	*Coartem, Riamet*	Novartis
	malathion	*Ovide*	Taro
	mebendazole	generics	
	mefloquine	generics	
§	meglumine antimonate	*Glucantime*	Sanofi, France
†	melarsoprol	*Mel-B*	
	metronidazole	*Flagyl*, generics	Pfizer
§	miconazole	*Monistat*	
†	miltefosine[1]	*Impavido, Miltex*	Paladin, Canada
§	niclosamide	*Yomesan*	
†	nifurtimox	*Lampit*	Bayer HealthCare
	nitazoxanide	*Alinia*	Romark
§	ornidazole	*Tiberal*	
§	oxamniquine	*Vansil, Mansil*	Pfizer, UK
	paromomycin	Oral: generics §Topical: *Leshcutan*	Sun Pharma

	pentamidine isethionate	*Pentam 300, NebuPent*	APP Pharmaceuticals
	permethrin	*Nix*	Insight, Bayer
	Elimite, generics	Renaissance Pharma	
	piperaquine/dihydroartemisin	*Euratesim*	Sigma Tau, Italy
	praziquantel	*Biltricide*	Bayer
	primaquine phosphate USP		Sanofi
§	proguanil	*Paludrine*	
	proguanil/atovaquone	*Malarone*	GlaxoSmithKline
§	propamidine isethionate	*Brolene*	Aventis
	pyrantel pamoate	*Pin-X, Reese's Pinworm*	Penn Labs, Reese
	pyrethrins and piperonyl butoxide	*Rid*	Bayer
§	pyrimethamine USP	*Daraprim*	Amedra
	quinidine gluconate	generics	
§	quinine dihydrochloride		
	quinine sulfate	*Qualaquin*	AR Scientific
	rifampin	*Rifadin*	Sanofi
†	sodium stibogluconate	*Pentostam*	GlaxoSmithKline, UK
§	spiramycin	*Rovamycine*	Sanofi, France
	sulfadiazine	generics	
†	suramin sodium	*Germanin*	Bayer, Germany
	tinidazole	*Tindamax*	Mission
	trimethoprim/sulfamethoxazole (TMP/SMX)	*Bactrim*, generics	Sun Pharma
§	triclabendazole	*Egaten*	Novartis

Generic Name	Brand Name	Manufacturer
§ trimetrexate	*Neutrexin*	

§ Not available in the US; may be available through a compounding pharmacy such as Expert Compounding Pharmacy, 6744 Balboa Blvd, Lake Balboa, CA 91406 (800-247-9767) or Medical Center Pharmacy, New Haven, CT (203-688-7064). Other compounding pharmacies may be found through the National Association of Compounding Pharmacies (800-687-7850) or the Professional Compounding Centers of America (800-331-2498, www.pccarx.com).

† Available from the CDC Drug Service, Centers for Disease Control and Prevention, Atlanta, Georgia 30333; 404-639-3670 (evenings, weekends, or holidays: 770-488-7100; fax: 404-639-3717).

* Available through an Investigational New Drug (IND) request from the FDA. IND request paperwork is available through the CDC.

1. Available from the CDC for treatment of infections with free-living amebae; available from the manufacturer through an IND application from the FDA for treatment of other infections.

Index